IS YOUR LIFESTYLE KILLING YOU?

THE 8 SIMPLE STEPS FOR
LASTING WEIGHT LOSS
AND
OPTIMAL HEALTH

Dr. Karen Wolfe,
M.B.B.S., MA

The purpose of this book is to educate and inform. This is not intended for self-diagnosis or treatment. It is recommended that you seek advice from your personal physician or health care provider before beginning any nutritional program. The author and publishing company shall have neither liability nor responsibility to any person or entity with respect to loss, damage, or injury caused or alleged to be caused directly or indirectly by the information contained in this book.

Dr. Karen Wolfe.

M.B.B.S. (Sydney), MA (Counseling Psychology)

Dr. Karen is an author, entrepreneur, speaker, and certified coach with The Institute for Integrative Nutrition. She is the author of *Medicine from the Inside Out, Create the Body Your Soul Desires* and several CD's including *Visualizations for Healing* and *Glycemic Index Made Easy*. Dr. Karen co-created *The Conscious Body Method Coaching System* with Dr. Deborah Kern, Ph.D. which is used by many individuals and coaches nationwide.

In 2007, Karen received The Service and Leadership Circle Award from the National Wellness Institute for her outstanding contributions to the field of wellness. One of her great passions is to mentor others to build successful businesses in the wellness field and to support others in their quest for optimal health.

Born and raised in Sydney, Australia, Dr. Karen was a very successful competitive swimmer for many years. She went to Sydney University Medical School and graduated with a Bachelor of Medicine and Bachelor of Surgery (M.B.B.S.). She worked initially in Australia as a Family Physician followed by eight years as Medical Director of the Australian Government Health Service.

Dr. Karen moved to the United States in 1991 and completed a Masters Degree in Counseling Psychology from the National University in California in 1993. She is an international speaker on wellness and nutrition, and she frequently speaks at conferences and professional organizations throughout the USA and abroad.

Dr. Karen lives in Mission Viejo, California with her American husband Steve. She has three children and two spunky dogs. She enjoys physical fitness, hiking, travel, and having a good ol' Aussie barbie at home with friends and family. You can visit her at her website:

www.drkarenwolfe.org

RESEARCH AND TECHNICAL OVERSIGHT
Linda Roll

Linda teaches English and writing courses online and spends her free time with her husband and three children.

ILLUSTRATIONS
Trevor Morris

Trevor is a full-time student and the Tribeca Flashpoint Media Arts Academy in Chicago and part-time cinematographer and unicycling enthusiast.

SPECIAL RECOGNITION FOR EDITING
Kelsey Grace Wolfe

Full-time student at The University of Minnesota-Twin Cities College of Education and Human Development

COVER DESIGN
Bella Guzmán

Balla is Creative Director at *Highwire Creative*

2nd Printing 2013. Printed in the United States of America

Quantity discounts are available on bulk purchases of this book for educational purposes. For information, please contact Healing Quest Publishing at
info@drkarenwolfe.org

I dedicate this book to my mum Ellen, my sister Sue, my husband Steve and our three children, Steve, Kendall, and Kelsey.

A special thanks to Kelsey for editing the final version of the book during Spring Break in her Freshman college year. I am so proud of the young woman you have become and am delighted to witness your confidence and personal strength. I know you will be successful at whatever you decide to do! You give me faith in the future and I am so blessed and proud to be your mom.

Contents

Introduction

Weighty Matters

The Price We Pay for the Lifestyles We Live

Our Killer Lifestyles

The Process to Recovery

The Healthy Lifestyle Solution

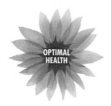

Introduction

Never doubt that a small group of thoughtful,
committed citizens can change the world.

- Margaret Mead

I agree wholeheartedly with Margaret Mead, and this book is my sincere effort to attract people who are properly informed about and committed to their own health and happiness in hopes that we can change the world. Ours is a daunting task but worthwhile nonetheless. It is a movement our world must embrace for its well-being.

The title, *Is Your Lifestyle Killing You,* may have startled you. That is intentional. The *New Merriam-Webster Dictionary* defines kill as "to put an end to" or "to deprive of life." That is exactly what is happening with many people as a result of their lifestyles.

This book will help you understand the underlying causes of almost any chronic health problem and weight issue. As I write this book, an epidemic of global proportions threatens our health and our happiness. This epidemic is not of an acute infectious type, but of a chronic, degenerative nature that plagues more and more of us each day. This epidemic grows steadily and influences every aspect of our health.

When our health is compromised, so is our happiness. According to the preliminary data for the *National Vital Statistics Report*, the 10 major causes of death in the United States in 2011 were as follows:

1. Heart Disease
2. Cancer
3. Chronic lung disease
4. Stroke
5. Accidents
6. Alzheimer's disease
7. Diabetes mellitus
8. Influenza/pneumonia
9. Kidney disease
10. Intentional self-harm

You'll notice that most causes of death are of a chronic nature. The trend in all developing nations is the same. More and more, the major causes of death worldwide are chronic, degenerative disease.

If we look at similar statistics for major causes of death from a century ago, we'll find a different story. The three main causes of death in 1900 were acute infections: pneumonia, tuberculosis, and diarrhea. The medical profession has curtailed these types of deaths. Nine-ty-seven years later, the major causes of death were heart disease, cancer, and stroke. Even more so today, the major health threats we face are chronic, degenerative diseases.

The following graphs come from an article published at *cdc.gov* (Centers for Disease Control and Prevention). They list the ten leading causes of death for both 1900 and 1997 respectively.

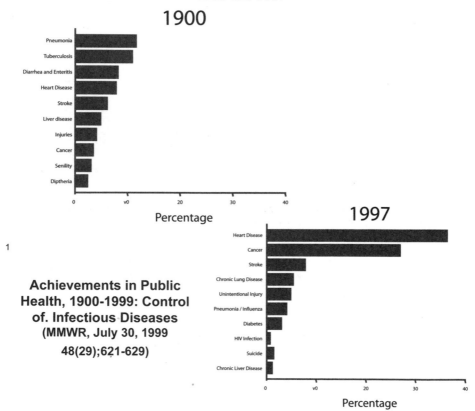

Leading Causes of Death as a Percentage of All Deaths
1900 and 1997

1

Achievements in Public Health, 1900-1999: Control of. Infectious Diseases
(MMWR, July 30, 1999
48(29);621-629)

---

1   For more information on the advancements in health in the last century, read the article Achievements in public health, 1900-1999: Control of infectious diseases at cdc.gov.

Obesity is the epidemic that impacts nearly all of these major threats to our health. As you look around, you can see that we are an overweight people. As a nation and a world, we are gaining stubborn weight that stays around and often refuses to go. Obesity itself is a risk factor in nearly every chronic illness that looms on the horizon. This collective weight is the price we pay for our modern lifestyles.

Excess weight is a natural consequence of the habits we have developed as part of our current way-of-life. You cannot separate the consequence from the action. It is time to discuss the actions that are steadily increasing our weight and decreasing our ability to live as we would choose to live.

Is this Book for You?

You may be thinking, "I'm not obese, so it's not my problem." You may be thinking, "My children are not obese, so it is not my problem." I'm here to tell you that, unfortunately, more than one out of every three people in the United States is obese. According to *Overweight and Obesity: Facts at the Centers for Disease Control and Prevention*, seventeen percent of our children are obese. The number increases dramatically if we include those who are overweight but not obese.

In the past 20 years, the amount of the population that is obese has increased substantially and the trend continues. Statistics show that, although it may not be your problem today, it is likely to be your problem one day in the future.

Although the US has the highest rates of obesity among its citizens, obesity is not just an American problem. The Organization for Economic Co-operation and Development (OECD), concluded:

> *Obesity has risen to the top of the public health policy agenda worldwide. Before 1980, rates were generally well below 10%. They have since doubled or tripled in many countries, and in almost half of the OECD, 50% or more of the population is overweight. A key risk factor for numerous chronic diseases, obesity is a major public health concern.*
>
> ("Obesity and the Economics of Prevention," 2010)

The real tragedy is that this global epidemic is largely brought on by lifestyle. Many, if not all, of the contributing factors to obesity and chronic illness are lifestyle choices. It is both wonderful and frightening. It is wonderful that we can influence our own health but frightening that so few of us do so.

Being trained as a doctor in the medical field, I see firsthand the disparity between western healthcare and true wellness. Medicine, as practiced in most developed countries, treats and manages disease. Thus, the healthcare system, in all reality, is more like a disease-care system. Lifestyle choices, that can make all the difference in the case of obesity and chronic illness such as type 2 diabetes, are rarely discussed. When they are discussed, it often comes after the diagnosis.

As a medical student and as a practicing physician, I felt this disease-centered approach did not focus enough on the true causes of disease. I wanted to teach my patients how to create wellness. That is why I wrote this book. We cannot wait for the healthcare system to change. We have to take action in our own lives and communities.

My life-long interest in health and wellness was not satisfied through my medical training. Please understand, I embrace and respect the advances of modern medicine. I acknowledge and celebrate its victories over pain, suffering, and disease. But I must be honest with myself and with you about its limitations. It doesn't take a medical degree or CDC statistics to know that modern medicine, although effective in arresting disease, does not focus enough on wellness.

I believe my own story is, in part, the story of us all. It is the joy of finding a solution that compelled me to write this book. Let me take you through the steps that led me to where I am today—a thoughtful, committed person determined to provide a solution to the epidemic of poor health and elusive happiness.

My Story

My interest in wellness developed early. I swam competitively and trained with the most prestigious swim team in Australia. Although my swimming career ended due to a shoulder injury, my interest in health and nutrition continued. With a desire to make wellness my career, I enrolled in medical school. I learned that the medical profession was less about wellness and more about disease management.

My disappointment subsided when I was asked to participate on panels designed to study the aging population in my native Australia. I was a Medical Officer with the Australian Government, and worked in many "think tanks" designed to create individual, community, and government solutions to the chronic disease epidemic that Australia faced at that time. I enjoyed being part of creating solutions based on examining true causes of illness.

After eight years in the Australian medical field, I left my homeland for love. Love brought me to the United States in the early 90s. Living in California opened doors for me to follow my heart and pursue a career in the wellness industry. With the help of a great mentor, I began speaking about health and wellness. I completed a Masters Degree in psychology that emphasized the effect of the mind on the body and wellness. I began coaching and mentoring others as they pursued a healthier and happier lifestyle.

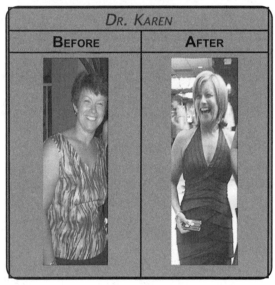

My journey was a personal one. I learned first-hand that my own lifestyle wasn't what it should be. For instance, I learned I was not eating as well as I had thought. I was dedicated to exercise, yet I was not experiencing optimal health. As I really began understanding the impact my daily habits had on my overall health and well-being, I made positive changes in my own lifestyle. I was thrilled to help others understand the connection between their choices and their health. I am happy to say I don't ask my clients to do anything that I have not done or to change anything that I have not changed in my own life.

This book is the culmination of my journey: eight years practicing medicine followed by twenty years speaking, coaching, and mentoring in the wellness industry. My journey has led me to a place where health and happiness are not only possible but enjoyed daily. I have come to understand that the choices I make each day shape my health and happiness today and tomorrow.

There is an answer to our global epidemic and it lies in these simple choices made each day. Wellness does not just happen. It will take a concentrated effort of "thoughtful, committed citizens" to focus on the lifestyle factors to solve our health crisis. I see myself as a change agent, and I am inviting you to join me by learning about wellness and placing yourself on your own path to health and happiness.

I want to share with you the tools and the knowledge I have gained over the past three decades to help you take the necessary steps to place you on that path. The method I will share with you is the same method I have used to experience a new level of wellness in my own life. I have trained and coached others in this method, and they too have experienced true wellness.

References

Hoyert, D. L., & Xu, J. US Department of Health and Human Services, Centers for Disease Control and Prevention. (2012). Deaths: Preliminary data for 2011 (National Vital Statistics Report Vol. 61 Num. 6). Retrieved from website: http://www.cdc.gov/nchs/data/nvsr/nvsr61/nvsr61_06.pdf

Obesity and the economics of prevention: Fit not fat. (2010, Sept 23). Retrieved from http://www.oecd.org/health/health-systems/obesityandtheeconomic-sofpreventionfitnotfat.htm

Overweight and obesity: Facts. (2012, April 27). Retrieved from http://www.cdc.gov/obesity/data/facts.html

US Department of Health and Human Services, Centers for Disease Control and Prevention. (1999). Achievements in public health, 1900-1999: Control of infectious diseases (Morbidity and Mortality Weekly Report 48(29);621-629). Retrieved from website: http://www.cdc.gov/mmwr/preview/mmwrhtml/mm4829a1.htm

Chapter 1

Weighty Matters

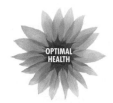

None knows the weight of another's burden.

- George Herbert

Weight is a burden many of us carry. It is the elephant on our backs. We gain and retain weight despite our best efforts to the contrary. I have certainly lost and re-gained the same ten pounds many times.

Although it seems a trivial thing, our weight often contributes significantly to our overall well-being both emotionally and physically. If you spend countless hours thinking about weight loss and talking about your weight, your diet, your disappointment, and your frustration, you are not alone.

Ours is a world obsessed with weight and weight loss. Rebecca Reinser, editor of *BusinessWeek.com,* estimates that Americans spend upwards of $40 billion yearly on diet products. More and more countries are similarly obsessed with dieting. The weight loss, or diet industry, grows each year as our preoccupation with weight increases.

There is no shortage of late-night infomercials touting the latest diet craze. You've seen them. "Lose ten pounds without doing a thing. Just take this little pill and the pounds will melt away." The words "fad diet" are now as much a part of our vocabulary and global conversation as the word diet itself. We are highly skeptical of any "diet" that comes along. Most of us know that what sounds like a miracle cure for that extra twenty pounds around the waist is likely just a passing craze.

Are you tired of fad diets that don't work? Do you feel that you have no willpower or self-discipline? Do you feel you've tried every diet and now have just given up the struggle? Does focusing on your weight occupy too much of your thoughts and attention? You are not alone.

And it isn't just dieting and losing weight that attract our attention and our wallet.

For each fad diet, there is an equal faddish exercise contraption designed to give maximum output with minimal effort. "Just thirty minutes a day and you'll have the body of your dreams." We've learned that without pain there is no gain, to use a common phrase.

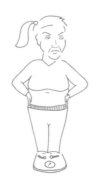 And so we turn to the pain—exercise. Sometimes we opt to exercise twice as hard and twice as much because dieting doesn't seem to work for us.

We fall into the cycle of diet and exercise . . . exercise and diet. Both honest and dishonest advertisements bombard us daily about the impact of diet and exercise on our weight. Our national and global obsession with weight is based largely on the physical aspect of it and the disgust we are trained to feel at the word 'overweight.' Weight contributes to our body image: the way we view ourselves. Weight is often the primary reason we are dissatisfied with our looks. For most of us, being overweight contributes to our unhappiness with our bodies more than any other factor.

Personally, I struggled with body image issues for most of my life. It started at age 10 when I became a competitive swimmer. There was so much pressure to be a certain weight. I was weighed each morning at swim practice. Because I was "chunkier" than the other swimmers, my coach would often make a derogatory comment about my weight. Even my log book where I kept track of the miles I swam every day had comments about my weight being a problem. I was so young and so impressionable. These ongoing comments from my coach began what I call my bad body thoughts. They occupied so much of my mental energy. For the next twenty or more years these bad body thoughts prevented me from truly living and loving life.

I hear similar stories daily from clients who are rebuilding their bodies (and their lives). Regina's story is such an inspiration, and I am glad she wanted to share it with you.

> *I didn't eat a lot of food yet no matter how little I ate, I just couldn't lose the weight.*

My self-esteem was in the garbage. I didn't even want to go out in public. I struggled with my weight since the birth of my son and was in even more trouble after the birth of my daughter. My cholesterol, LDL, and triglycerides were all high for the first time ever. I was desperate to lose weight, be healthy, and get my life back.

The more weight I gained, the less activities I wanted to or could do. I even struggled climbing stairs and doing basic routines. I had to find out what was wrong with me. Only now do I realize that I was eating high-glycemic meals and had become insulin resistant.

By using Dr. Karen's program, I have now lost a total of 46 pounds and 3 sizes in under 7 months! I feel dramatically better mentally and physically. My energy levels are up as well as my confidence and self-esteem. I even roller-skated for the first time in years. Everyday I think about how awesome it feels to be able to move around with little effort and without feeling tired.

I follow The Healthy Lifestyle Solution. My eating habits are totally different, and I do not crave processed foods anymore. I feel healthier and know my body gets what it needs. I had my blood work done after 6 months of being on the program, and I cannot believe the results below!

Regina's Healthy Lifestyle Solution 6 Month Scores			
Measurement	*July*	*6 mo. later*	*Change*
Total Cholesterol	244	204	▼ 40
Triglycerides	149	81	▼ 68
LDL	156	127	▼ 29
HDL (good)	58	59	▲ 1

This program works and is very easy to follow. I have personally grown and learned so much in these last months.

Regina R., Denver

For many of us, weight literally becomes a burden we carry each day of our lives. It weighs us down and depresses our spirits. Weight loss is the battle in which we have surrendered. We've thrown up our hands and given up the fight. The path is too hard and too long. The rewards are too few and too costly. We shrug our shoulders and resign ourselves to our fate—too much weight and not enough will power.

Beyond Physical Weight

Ironically, we expend too much time and energy concerned about the cosmetic aspects of weight and too little time and energy concerned about how our weight actually impacts our health and what it means for our future. It is easy to focus on the physical nature of weight because we see it and live it daily. However, our weight impacts our body systems resulting in devastating effects. The dire consequences of our weight are more than skin deep and are often hidden from our immediate view.

It is so easy to overlook how our weight may be impacting our health on the inside. Yet it is precisely what is happening inside that truly matters and leads to what we see on the outside. If we could be more motivated to care for our internal well-being, the outer appearance would improve by default. Releasing weight results from taking better care of the inner self.

The medical profession, wellness coaches, and the public at large are 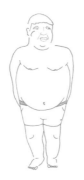 beginning to understand the impact of weight on our health. Being overweight, like smoking, increases a person's risk for most chronic and degenerative diseases. Let's take a moment to understand what we mean when we say chronic and degenerative.

Although we are living longer than our predecessors, we are also dying longer. The diseases that plague mankind today are of a chronic nature. They come on gradually and linger for years if not for a lifetime. Degeneration is the deterioration of our body over time. Degenerative disease slowly and consistently eats away at our health. These diseases include type 2 diabetes, heart disease, cancer, high blood pressure, and arthritis to name only a few.

The Global Epidemic: Obesity

Where does all this talk of weight and disease lead us? It leads us to a discussion about the global epidemic that is obesity. We are facing an obesity and chronic disease crisis worldwide that affects adults and children alike. Despite the trillions expended on health care worldwide, we as a world seem to be experiencing more disease and more sickness rather than less. While it is true that obesity rates in the US are higher than most other countries, it is also true that obesity poses a problem for most developed countries.

The OECD, you'll remember, recognizes obesity as a "major public health concern" because it is a key risk factor for numerous chronic diseases ("Obesity and the," 2010). The CDC claims that overweight and obesity-related medical conditions are the second leading cause of preventable death in the US ("Adult obesity facts," 2012). Let me repeat that. These conditions can be prevented.

Obesity and Diabetes

As we discuss obesity and its influence on our health or lack thereof, let's focus on type 2 diabetes to illustrate my point. According to the International Diabetes Federation (IDF), 371 million people worldwide have diabetes and the number of diabetics is on the rise in every country. The IDF projects that diabetes will affect nearly 552 million by the year 2030. The IDF reports on seven regions, and each region has staggering statistics. In North America and the Caribbean, one in ten adults has diabetes. The Western Pacific region has the largest number of diabetics. One-fifth of adults with diabetes live in the South-East Asia region ("Idf diabetes atlas, 2012").

This is not just an American epidemic. In 2010, I spoke at a conference in Saudi Arabia on the topic of type 2 diabetes. It was then that I learned how widespread diabetes is. The Middle East has one of the highest percentages of the population with diabetes. Between 2011 and 2030, there is projected to be a 51% increase in numbers of adults with diabetes worldwide ("Idf diabetes atlas, 2012").

The correlation between weight and diabetes is unmistakable. Research shows that weight can be a major contributing factor to the onset of type 2 diabetes. An article, published in *Diabetes Care*, concluded that even a 7% weight loss could produce as much as a 58% improvement in the risk of progressing from prediabetes to diabetes ("The diabetes prevention," 2002).

What is true of type 2 diabetes is also true of many chronic, degenerative diseases. To some degree or another, they are preventable. The Center for Disease Control says behavior, environment, and genetic factors all contribute to obesity ("Adult obesity facts," 2012). The same may be said of heart disease, cancer, Alzheimer's, or any other chronic illness. We will address environmental and genetic factors later, but let's focus for now on lifestyle.

Lifestyle is a catch-all phrase that refers to our diet, exercise, sleep habits, stress, and other factors. Suffice it to say, our diets and our exercise habits can play a significant role in reducing our risk of developing the aforementioned conditions.

Most of us know that we should eat healthy food and exercise, but the way we understand "healthy" may not be accurate and most of us certainly don't understand what happens inside the body when food, good or bad, enters our system. I want to help you understand what is happening to your body and why previous attempts at releasing weight may have failed.

I return to my clients for an example. Terry is a registered nurse with an RN and BSN. After she worked with me, using the program I will share with you in this book, Terry was able to look back at her lifestyle habits before she began the program. This is what she said upon reflection

> *Thank you so much for your help. It seems no one could figure out why I never lost weight even with all the activity and exercise in addition to trying to eat well. Even though I ate somewhat well, I now know that I truly was addicted (to sugar).*

Here is Terry's letter to me in full.

> *Dr. Karen,*
>
> *I am so pleased to tell you I am releasing weight on the program. I think this will help me obtain the lifestyle I so desire. Thank you so much for your help. It seems no one could figure out why I never lost weight even with a lot of activity and exercise and trying to eat well. Even though I ate somewhat well, I now know that I ate too many carbs and truly was addicted.*
>
> *Thank you for saving my life for meaningful happiness. I think probably the carbs over the years have taken their toll.*
>
> *Terry M., RN, BSN, North Carolina*

Willpower is NOT Enough

It is time to really unleash the key to how our bodies work. Most people think that calories in and calories out are the only things that determine whether we release weight, gain weight, or stay the same.

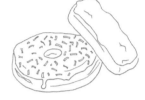

Although this is an important consideration, our bodies are much more complex than that. Here is the message that most of us never hear, yet it is the beginning of a whole new freedom from weight battles.

The Power of Brain Chemistry

Self-care starts with learning about your
physiology - more specifically, your brain.
— Dr. Joel Robertson

I have worked in the Wellness Industry for over 20 years, but a major shift in my effectiveness as a wellness coach happened about ten years ago. I attended a conference in Anaheim, California and heard Dr. Joel Robertson speak. He opened my eyes to a critical piece of the puzzle of health.

In his book, *Peak Performance Living - Easy, Drug-Free Ways to Alter Your Own Brain Chemistry* (1996), Dr. Robertson writes:

I have rarely met a person who was overweight or stressed . . who didn't know what their problems were. But changing their behavior is difficult for most people. Contrary to my education, I concluded that such people aren't noncompliant and unwilling or unmotivated, but that the solutions professionals provide for them are inconsistent with their brain chemical reward system.

The impact of our brain chemistry can't be ignored in a discussion about health. The brain and its functions play a significant role in our ability to care for ourselves.

Brain Chemistry 101

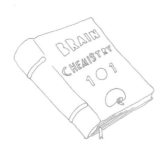

It was Joel Robertson's lecture many years ago where I learned that, whether we know it or not, we are altering our brain chemistry constantly through what we eat, how we exercise, how we sleep, and how we think. All our behaviors create neuro-chemical changes in the body.

I am going to take you on a little journey to explain, in simple terms, the mechanism be-hind how this occurs and why it is important. I know this is a lot of science, but every time I speak about this in a lecture, my audience members tell me how helpful it is. I wanted to make sure I shared it here.

Neurotransmitters and Lifestyle

There are a powerful group of chemicals inside the brain (and body) called neurotransmitters. Neurotransmitters create a wide spectrum of feelings, moods, and thoughts. They can affect everything from feelings of self-confidence and self-esteem to enhanced memory and deep sleep.

During the past thirty years, science has learned that neurotransmitters can be affected, often dramatically, by a wide variety of everyday behaviors. One of the most powerful is the food we eat.

The fact is we have more power than we realize to shape our inner world. Most of us manipulate our brain biochemistry and "inner world" unconsciously. I know this first hand.

Over and over, my "automatic behavior" reaches for my "comfort food" to ease stress, only to pay the price later of a dull mind, low energy, regret and self-loathing.

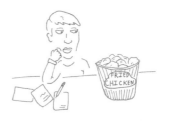

We often use food to deal with stress and emotional pain. Unfortunately, most of us manipulate our brain chemistry badly.

Each of us needs to be aware of the adverse effects of modern life on the body. The stresses of modern life, which are unlike any other in previous human experience, are causing aberrations in body biochemistry and human behavior.

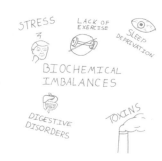

Our biochemistry is progressively changed by the changes in the way we eat, the way we work, and the way we live.

IN A NUTSHELL

Specific neurotransmitters are highly sensitive to the foods we consume and actually play a major role in how our bodies respond to our diet. Physicians often prescribe medicines that are, in reality, a manipulation of neurotransmitters in order to alleviate depression, anxiety, and other mood disorders. Our behavior, our lifestyle, and our relationship with food are interrelated.

Many people today suffer from imbalances in brain and body chemistry because of the standard Western diet, our sedentary lifestyles, the pressures of time, and the continual bombardment of stimuli in the media. All of these "lifestyle factors" combine to create biochemistry imbalances, and these imbalances distort our behavior.

The Informational Network

Another way to understand this is to imagine the body as an informational network made up of billions of cells that talk to each other. These cells do not actually touch each other. Rather, there is a tiny space between the cells called a *synaptic gap*. The neurotransmitters, or the chemical messengers, pass information across this space.

At any given time, there can be a sufficiency of a certain neurotransmitter, a deficiency of a certain neurotransmitter, or a dominance of a certain neurotransmitter. We can have too much, too little, or just the right amount of each neurotransmitter at any given moment.

Therefore, our brain chemistry profile constantly changes. It fluctuates moment to moment depending on the food we choose to eat, the stress we feel, the sleep we get, the exercise we do, and so on. The good news—we can manipulate our diets and other lifestyle choices to balance our brain chemistry and, ultimately, improve our health.

Are you still with me? Trust me, this information will really help you.

Brain Chemistry and Cravings

There are many problems that may arise from chemical imbalances in the brain. One that is less often recognized and most often lived is the development of cravings. I'd like to spend some time discussing cravings in light of brain chemistry and chemical imbalance.

Many different lifestyle factors contribute to cravings. This is brain chemistry in action because a brain chemistry imbalance is often signaled by a craving. In other words, the body detects it is lacking something and sends a signal to alert the body to fill that need.

Ideally, the body should be able to detect the need, send the signal, fulfill the need (often in the form of food), and satisfy the craving. The simplest example might be water. Have you ever craved water? When we exercise or spend time in the sun, our bodies need more water to compensate for the loss of water through exertion or heat. Our bodies will cause us to crave water to ensure that the need is filled.

Unfortunately, when our bodies experience imbalances in the bio-chemistry of the brain, the system of craving can work against us rather than in our favor.

The Unsweetened Facts behind our Craving Nation

If we are out of balance, what we crave can keep us further out of balance. I experience this often in my own life. When I travel, am sleep-deprived, and working long hours, I notice my cravings creeping back. (They certainly aren't cravings for broccoli and green beans). The stress of travel triggers my sugar cravings.

Eating my favorite sugar, black licorice, would not be the healthiest action for me to take to restore balance. Foods high in sugar do not restore balance, but create more imbalance by increasing blood sugar levels. The fact is, giving into my sugar cravings makes me feel worse. I suffer consequences of tiredness, lethargy, irritability, and lack of concentration. I've learned to use that craving signal as a message to me to slow down and practice good self-care. The chart below is an example of how our blood sugar affects so many aspects of our lives. I use this chart all the time as a barometer of how balanced I am.

Balancing Blood Sugar	
Balanced Blood Sugar	**Unbalanced Blood Sugar**
Energetic	Tired all the time
Tired when appropriate	Tired for no reason
Focused and relaxed	Restless, can't keep still
Clear	Confused
Having a good memory	Having trouble remembering
Able to concentrate	Having trouble concentrating
Can solve problems effectively	Easily frustrated
Easygoing	More irritable than usual
Even-tempered	Getting angry unexpectedly

Addressing Brain Chemistry to Improve Health

When you recognize an imbalance, it is possible to use food and supplementation safely to support the increase of specific neurotransmitters and restore balance. Our brains use more than a dozen neurotransmitters, but we'll focus on one that I talk about all the time. It has a powerful effect on our moods and behavior and can be manipulated by daily behavior. It is serotonin.

Serotonin: What It Does

Serotonin is one of the relaxing chemicals in the brain. People with sufficient serotonin levels experience happiness with themselves and their surroundings. They feel appreciation, confidence, and a general sense of well-being and contentment.

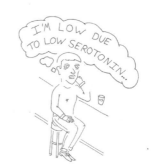

When serotonin levels are low, you may feel depressed, act impulsively, and have intense cravings for alcohol, sweets, or carbohydrates. You may feel unsatisfied if starch is not part of your meal and you may struggle more than others if you attempt a low carbohydrate diet. This may trigger a depression that can manifest may result in weight gain, insatiable cravings for carbs, and/or a general pessimistic attitude.

Serotonin Level Effects	
Optimal Level of Serotonin	**Low Level of Serotonin**
Hopeful, optimistic	Depressed
Reflective and thoughtful	Impulsive
Able to concentrate	Having short attention span
Creative, focused	Blocked, scattered
Able to think things through	Flying off the handle
Able to seek help	Suicidal
Responsive	Reactive
Looking forward to dessert without an emotional charge	Craving sweets
Hungry for a variety of different foods	Craving mostly carbohydrates like bread, pasta and cereal

How Food Affects Serotonin Levels

Serotonin is made from the amino acid tryptophan. Tryptophan comes from the protein you eat during the day. But having tryptophan available to make serotonin requires more than simply eating foods that contain it.

Dr. Kathleen DesMaisons, Ph.D. is the one who first who alerted me to the powerful role serotonin plays in cravings. Her work has made a huge impact on my life personally and professionally. I highly recommend her book *Potatoes Not Prozac*. She is a colleague and a friend, and she is so masterful at explaining how eating the right food at the right time can balance your neurochemistry. With her permission, I have an excerpt from her book, *Potatoes Not Prozac*, to explain a very important way food affects serotonin levels.

BLOOD/BRAIN BARRIER

PROTEIN TRYPTOPHAN SEROTONIN

After you eat protein, your body breaks it down into different amino acids. These amino acids travel to the brain in your bloodstream, but they cannot immediately

*enter your brain cells because there is a blood-brain barrier that
controls what can enter your brain cells.*

*Tryptophan swims up to the blood-brain barrier with all the other amino acids. But there are far fewer tryptophan molecules
than these other amino acid molecules. In fact, tryptophan is
outnumbered and loses out in the competition to cross the
brain cell blood-brain barrier. Think of tryptophan as a runt that
gets left behind in the shuffle. This means that eating protein
with high levels of tryptophan alone won't work. The runt
needs help!*

*Your body has a special way to help this runt get across the
blood-brain barrier. When the body releases insulin, the insulin
seeks out amino acids to use for building muscle. But insulin is
not interested in our runt (tryptophan). It wants only the big guys.
So, it carries off the other amino acids to other parts of the body
where muscle can be found, leaving little tryptophan behind.
This is good, for now tryptophan can hop across the blood-brain
barrier and be put to use making serotonin. And more serotonin
makes you feel better (144-145).*

Naturally Increase Serotonin Levels

Modern living takes a costly toll on our health. Irregular sleep patterns,
processed foods, a sedentary lifestyle, even
the air we breathe are serious factors in the
depletion of the body's serotonin system.
Under stress, serotonin levels can plummet,
so the body starts to crave simple carbohydrates to give us a boost of insulin.

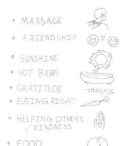

Isn't it amazing that our daily activities create
changes in our neurochemistry? Walking in
the park or in nature, stretching exercises,
gentle yoga poses, reading and meditation
can promote the production of serotonin.

The feeling from these kinds of activities are peaceful, quieting, reflec-
tive, and meditative. At the same time, your inner emotional state is
elevated by the increasing levels of serotonin being produced. Thus
you have set up a positive cycle in which exercise or relaxation boosts
serotonin, and this serotonin boosts mood.

Here are some of my favorite serotonin-boosting foods:

Dr. Karen's favorite serotonin-boosting foods

- Nuts
- Grilled chicken breast
- Peanut butter
- Greek yogurt
- Quinoa

- Egg whites
- Tuna
- Turkey
- Cottage cheese
- Salmon

Sugar and Food Addiction – Just Say No?

Now that we understand more of how our diets affect our brain chemistry, let's discuss addiction. I do not believe any discussion of weight is complete unless we address the psychology of eating and addiction.

Addiction is needing a substance, or believing we need a substance, whether or not that substance is beneficial to our bodies. We usually associate addiction with drugs like alcohol, marijuana, or nicotine. Less understood is food addiction. Through our dietary habits and other lifestyle factors, we can develop a dependency on food that sabotages our efforts to control our weight.

When I coach someone, I start by explaining that food is a drug and can be highly potent and addictive. Why is it so hard for us to lose weight despite the social stigma and health consequences being overweight brings? It is not because we want to be fat. It is partly because certain types of food are addictive. When we understand that food is a drug, we can manipulate it for positive results.

Jennifer's story is a powerful one and I am delighted that she agreed to share it here with us.

> *I am living proof that anything is possible. One day I decided "THIS IS IT" I want more out of life. I transformed myself from a fatigued, procrastinator and sugar junky with low self-esteem to a woman with the confidence to honor who I want to be physically and emotionally.*
>
> *My journey began with the 5 Day Sugar Cleanse and Dr. Karen's Sugar Buster Program. I was surprised in five days I lost four pounds and reduced my sugar cravings. The Sugar Buster calls*

helped me recognize what I was doing wrong and easy ways to make adjustments that fit my busy lifestyle.

I still use the knowledge I learned from the calls to empower me when I want to give up. I'm still learning. Today I am proud to uncover the physical body I knew awaited me along with an open mind that I am the creator of my destiny. As a single mom sometimes it can be tough but the alternative feels worse.

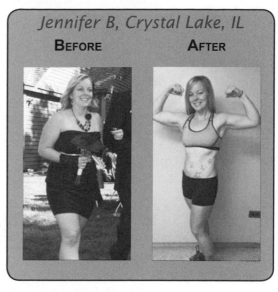

Jennifer B, Crystal Lake, IL
BEFORE   AFTER

I MAKE time to move my body and have an abundance of energy. I teach my daughter the importance of eating healthy to keep us strong and healthy.

- Jennifer B, Crystal Lake, IL

In my work with the Institute for Integrative Nutrition, I studied all of the dietary theories. One that truly resonates with me is Michael Pollan's theory. In his book, *In Defense of Food*, he explains that food that is made in a plant rather than grown on a plant can be biologically addictive.

What Pollan means is that when food is processed in a manufacturing facility, it is more likely to be addictive than food that is consumed in its natural state. He believes there are biological mechanisms that drive food addiction, and that certain types of food are addictive.

In the case of addiction, willpower is just not enough. Have you ever tried to give up your Coke or Mountain Dew? Sugar sweetened drinks are some of the most addictive agents. My client, Denise, learned she was addicted to diet soda and she wrote me this letter.

Before the program, I drank Diet Coke every day and since I started I quit cold turkey. For me, it is better not to have any because then I will want more. While I felt I ate healthy foods before this program, I realize now that I ate foods (bread/potatoes) that

*spiked my blood sugar levels. I ate more, was hungry more
often, and was tired and fatigued. I realized I am carbohydrate
sensitive. I know that my weakness is bread and potatoes.*

*This program is a lifestyle change. I know I will be tempted and
will probably fall down, but I know how to redirect and focus
myself again. My goal is not to beat myself up over it. We are only
human. The nice part is the flexibility. You get to choose what is
convenient for you.*

Denise, MD

Science now explains that we can, in fact, be biologically addicted to
sugar in the same way we can be addicted to heroin, cocaine, or
nicotine *Neuroscience & Biobehavioral Reviews* (Avena, Rade, Hoebel, 2008).
Binge-eating and other addictive behaviors are similar in both alcohol-
ics and sugar addicts. In fact, one study found that sugar can be even
more addictive than cocaine.

Lenore, Serre, and Cantin discovered that
sugar surpasses what is called "cocaine
reward" (2007). It is hard to think of sugar as
an addictive substance. Your child's favorite
treat and your "guilty pleasure" may, in fact,
be the most consumed of all addictive sub-
stances.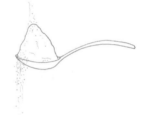

To say that Americans are on a sugar binge is
a dramatic *understatement*. According to one
article, "[In] the past 25 years, the average person's intake of sugar
and other natural sweeteners ballooned from 123 to as many as 160
pounds a year" *(Guthrie, 2006)*. We are consuming such large amounts
of sugar that it is no wonder we are bogged down by our weight. And
the worst part is we often consume sugar without realizing how much
has been added to the foods we eat.

Refined sugar isn't just in candy and ice cream. The processed foods
we rely on are laden with sugar. It becomes such a habit, we eat
these processed foods unaware of the damage we are inflicting on
our bodies. Eating highly-processed foods filled with sugar sets up
a vicious cycle that results in nutritional deficiencies and leads to the
chronic illness and obesity epidemic we've been discussing.

Do you remember the potato chip commercial that taunted us to try to eat just one? Well, I know I can't. When we eat low quality food—food that has been stripped of its natural content and filled up instead with additives and man-made sugars—we begin down the slippery slope of increased appetite, cravings, weight gain, and general dissatisfaction.

When we eat highly processed food, the body knows it is not satisfied and those cravings we talked about earlier develop. This leads to more physiological imbalance and more cravings. These foods we consume actually cause us to eat more.

It is important to note that long-term food addiction can begin in childhood. Well-intentioned mothers unknowingly assist in creating food addiction in their children. These moms slide the cereal off the shelf and fill up little Tommy's bowl before sending him off to school. Kids are actually beginning an addiction every morning from their cereal bowls.

Breakfast cereal is often made from wheat, coated in sugar, and then covered in milk. Like sugar, wheat and dairy have addictive properties. Like sugar, wheat and dairy activate pathways in the brain that signal pleasure and reward. Again, these are the same pathways that drugs like heroin or cocaine follow. I personally find it fascinating that food is a drug, yet we have ignored the biochemical impact for far too long.

HOW THE FOOD INDUSTRY DELIVERS HIGHLY ENGINEERED EATING EXPERIENCE ("EATERTAINMENT")

The advent of processed foods has dramatically altered the human diet, and we're now reaping the results in the form of rapidly rising chronic health problems. In his book, *The End of Overeating*, David Kessler, MD, the former head of the Food and Drug Administration, describes the science of how food is made into drugs by the creation of hyper-palatable foods that lead to neuro-chemical addiction. These foods trigger dopamine and serotonin in the body which sets up an addictive cycle (2009). The food industry knows how to manipulate foods for maximum chemical effect on the brain.

We are beginning to understand that our lifestyles and the thought process that brought us easy, fast, delectable, processed food needs to change. We know that the food companies are here to stay. Fast food restaurants and supermarkets are woven into the very fabric of American society. The change must begin with us. We have to become better educated about our food, where it comes from, and how it is made. We have to make informed, individual decisions about removing from our diets the dangerous, highly-processed foods we find in supermarkets and restaurants.

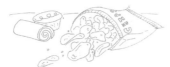

Every day I witness, in many of my clients, the effects of food as a drug. When that drug is altered, there are shifts in mood, energy, sleep habits, weight, concentration, and more. A client of mine, let's call her Susan, is an example of this.

Susan felt tired all the time and had constant carbohydrate cravings. No one could understand why she could never release weight even when she exercised consistently and ate well. That is, she thought that she was eating well.

Susan craved crackers, chips, bread, and other carbohydrates. She ate them even though she knew she shouldn't. It wasn't until she followed my low-refined-sugar eating plan, that she began to drop the pounds without feeling hungry or deprived. Susan's energy levels improved as did her confidence and self-esteem. She discovered she had been addicted to sugary, processed carbohydrates. She needed help to overcome that addiction, and I was able to offer her a food plan that worked.

There is a fundamental flaw in our current nutrition education. Just telling someone what to eat and what not to eat doesn't work because it ignores the fact that most of our commercially available food is highly addictive, and no matter how harmful a food or substance may be to the body, the sensation of pleasure keeps us coming back for more. The pleasure-seeking brain will always override the cognitive brain. We don't just tell an alcoholic to stop drinking. Likewise, we can't simply tell a food addict to stop eating.

I have observed sugar addiction while coaching my clients, and I've experienced it first-hand in my own life. Few of us are free from this addiction. We will continue to explore this topic throughout the book.

BRAIN BIOCHEMISTRY

FACT 1

Most behavior is unconscious, and we unconsciously change our brain chemistry all the time through our thoughts, behavior, and lifestyle choices.

FACT 2

Our "cravings" that drive us to eat, act, and think certain ways have biochemical drives that can reinforce more imbalance.

FACT 3

We can use this information by engaging in lifestyles that support a healthy biochemistry.

The Problem Explained

So by now you can see the problem of weight isn't simply a cosmetic one. Too much weight leads to obesity and chronic diseases such as diabetes. These conditions are manifestations of deeper problems inside the body and the brain.

We've discussed neurotransmitters and brain chemistry, which can lead us to destructive cravings and food addiction. Now let's turn to another internal problem, inflammation, which also contributes to the obesity and chronic disease epidemic we face today.

DR. KAREN'S TOP TEN TAKEAWAYS
FROM
WEIGHTY MATTERS

1. Our weight contributes to our overall well-being.

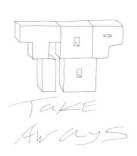

2. Weight can be a major factor to the onset of type 2 diabetes.

3. Our bodies are more complex than calories in/calories out.

4. Our behaviors create neurochemical changes in the body.

5. "Lifestyle factors" combine to create biochemistry imbalances.

6. Imbalances in the biochemistry of the brain can keep us out of balance.

7. We can manipulate our diets to balance brain chemistry.

8. It is possible to use food and supplementation safely to restore balance.

9. When we understand that food is a drug, we can manipulate it for positive results.

10. Just telling someone what to eat and what not to eat doesn't work.

CALL TO ACTION
WHAT YOU CAN DO!

• Recognize how you have moved away from supporting your physical, psychological and spiritual health.

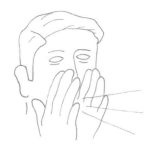

- Commit to taking one small step and share that commitment with a friend.

- Use any craving signal as a message to practice good self-care.

- Eat protein with every meal.

- Increase your intake of serotonin boosting foods.

- Remove sugar sweetened drinks from your diet.

- Remove diet drinks from your diet.

- Eliminate all artificial sweeteners from your diet for two weeks. (If you are skeptical, eliminate the sweeteners for two weeks. After two weeks of being artificial sweetener-free, reintroduce your artificial sweetener of choice in a significant quantity--about three servings daily--and notice how you feel compared to when you were consuming no artificial sweeteners).

- Use stevia, a safe, natural sweetener, as a substitute.

References

(2002). *The diabetes prevention program (dpp): Description of lifestyle intervention. Diabetes Care, 25(12),* 2165-2171. *Retrieved from http://care.diabetes-journals.org/content/25/12/2165.full.pdf*

Adult obesity facts. (2012, Aug). Retrieved from http://www.cdc.gov/obesity/data/adult.html

Avena, N. M., Rada, P., & Hoebel, B. G. (2008). Evidence for sugar addiction: Behavioral and neurochemical effects of intermittent, excessive sugar intake. Neuroscience & Biobehavioral Reviews, 32(1), 20-39. doi: 10.1016/j.neubiorev.2007.04.019

Centers for Medicare & Medicaid Services, Office of the Actuary, National Health Statistics Group. (n.d.). Retrieved from website: https://www.cms.gov/Research-Statistics-Data-and-Systems/Statistics-Trends-and-Reports/NationalHealthExpendData/Downloads/proj2010.pdf

DesMaisons, K. (2008). Potatoes not prozac. New York: Simon & Schuster.

Guthrie, C. (2006, August). Sugar breakdown. Experience Life, Retrieved from http://experiencelife.com/article/sugar-breakdown/

Hooper, J., & Teresi, D. (1986). The three-pound universe. New York: Macmillan.

Idf diabetes atlas update 2012. (n.d.). Retrieved from http://www.idf.org/diabetesatlas/5e/Update2012

Kessler, D. A. (2009). The end of overeating: taking control of the insatiable american appetite. New York: Macmillan.

Lenoir M, Serre F, Cantin L, Ahmed SH (2007) *Intense Sweetness Surpasses Cocaine Reward.* PLoS ONE 2(8): e698. doi:10.1371/journal.pone.0000698

Obesity and the economics of prevention: Fit not fat. (2010, Sept 23). Retrieved from http://www.oecd.org/health/health-systems/obesityandtheeconomic-sofpreventionfitnotfat.htm

Pollan, M. (2008). *In defense of food: an eater's manifesto.* New York: Penguin Press.

Reinser, R. (2008). *The diet industry: A big fat lie. BusinessWeek,* Retrieved from http://www.businessweek.com/deateroom/archives/2008/01/the_diet_in-dust.html

Robertson, J. C. (1996). *Peak performance living.* San Francisco: Harper.

Chapter 2

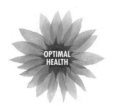

The Price We Pay
for the
Lifestyles We Live

Surgeons can cut out everything except cause.
- Herbert M. Shelton

It is time to delve into what is happening inside our bodies as a result of the lifestyles we live. Understanding this will open a new awareness of the link between healthy lifestyles, quality of life, and our health.

Inflammation: The Root of the Problem

Our bodies are amazingly complicated and yet incredibly simple. The body naturally protects itself from foreign invaders, be they infectious bacteria, harmful viruses, or environmental toxins. The body will attempt to protect and heal itself.

One naturally occurring immune response to injury is the process of inflammation. We've all experienced inflammation as we've cut ourselves shaving or sprained an ankle while exercising. When we get a cut, our bodies flood the area with immune response cells. We'll notice redness, pain, heat, and swelling. All of these are part of the inflammation response. The purpose is to heal the damaged area.

However, the old adage *too much of a good thing* fits inflammation perfectly. Although our bodies use inflammation as a natural defense mechanism against infection or injury, problems arise when harmful internal cellular damage consistently assail our bodies. The body, in turn, is in a state of perpetual inflammation. In fact, excess inflammation may be the highest price we pay for our killer lifestyles.

Inflammation, Obesity and Chronic Disease

Most people are ignorant to the role inflammation plays in this obesity and chronic disease epidemic we face. Yet understanding inflammation and its double-edged sword is crucial if we are going to positively impact these epidemics, our health, and our waist size.

For several years now, doctors and researchers have been learning about inflammation's role in determining our likelihood for developing the chronic diseases we'd all like to avoid. In fact, the biggest change I've seen in the medical field is the discovery that inflammation is a common denominator and root cause of many serious illnesses.

Whether we know it or not, inflammation touches every aspect of our health. Scientists have determined beyond doubt that inflammation is linked to heart disease, cancer, diabetes, rheumatoid arthritis, Alzheimer's, irritable bowel syndrome, and many other chronic, degenerative diseases.

Since inflammation underlies chronic disease, I'll spend some time exploring inflammation with you as it pertains to diet, weight, and age-related illness. Only through understanding are we equipped to combat the negative effects of inflammation, freeing our bodies from the destructive power of this innate and important immune reaction.

What exactly is Inflammation?

Inflammation comes from the Latin word *inflammo* which means 'I ignite' or 'I set aflame'. I like to refer to it as in-flame-ation. Inflammation is often characterized by the sensation of heat.

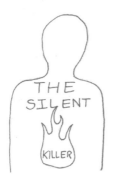

For instance, when our bodies are fighting the cold or flu virus, we often get a fever. We rush to treat the fever, but it actually indicates that the body is defending against the harmful substance encountered within. Another typical manifestation of inflammation is redness. When we cut ourselves shaving, as we mentioned earlier, the wound will appear red on the surface of the skin. Redness, like heat, points to the healing process. The redness lessens as the wound heals.

One of the more common symptoms of inflammation is swelling. When we sprain an ankle, for instance, it swells. Like the fever, we treat the swelling. However, the swelling is simply the body's way of protecting from further injury. A swollen ankle is painful and less mobile than a healthy ankle. Pain and restricted mobility complete the spectrum of the symptoms of inflammation.

Under normal conditions, inflammation helps the body rebound from injury and brings nourishment and more immune activity to the site of injury or infection. Our immune system is designed to defend and protect the body. Inflammation, as part of our immune response, is designed to promote healing for the benefit of the body.

Inflammation-Too Much of a Good Thing

Most of us only ever consider the inflammatory response as seen on the surface of the skin. But what about injury that occurs deep inside the body of which we are unaware? When our bodies are in a state contrary to a "healthy" state, the body unleashes immune responses of which inflammation is primary.

So you can probably now understand that many components of our killer lifestyle, such as processed food, toxic chemicals, and stress, can unleash a defensive immune response. Our bodies are so sophisticated that an increase in a hormone such as insulin can induce the inflammatory response. That sounds well and good, but an excess of the inflammatory response can be detrimental to our health.

> **INFLAMMATION AND DEPRESSION**
>
> Elevated levels of a substance called C-Reactive Protein (CRP) are a byproduct of inflammation in the body. Researchers have determined that high levels of CRP in the blood correspond with a higher risk of psychological stress and clinical depression, according to a *New York Times* article (Bakalar, 2012).

Hidden inflammation can trigger chronic disease and experts are just beginning to understand how stress, inactivity, exposure to toxins, and dietary choices fan the flame of inflammation inside the body. In other words, our lifestyle behaviors have a major impact on how much inflammation is happening in our bodies. When our lifestyle behaviors consistently "injure" the cells and functions of the body, we are in a state of chronic, low-grade inflammation. This chronic inflammation is now considered to play a causative role in the development of many chronic and degenerative diseases.

Let's discuss for a moment what perpetuates a state of chronic, hidden inflammation within our bodies. They are found in both our internal and our external environments. Many will come as no surprise as they have been occupying a spot on our New Year's resolution lists for decades now. This is not an exhaustive list nor does it appear in any particular order, but it does speak to the message of this book.

So what causes inflammation? Here are just a few of them:

- *Emotional Stress*: The stress we feel as a byproduct of living in the world today.
- *Physical Inactivity*: Our sedentary lives are catching up with us.
- *Environmental Allergens*: We are surrounded by them. Glues, adhesives, plastics, air fresheners, cleaning products — these are just some of the vast array of chemicals we are exposed to every day.
- *Sleep Deprivation*: Inadequate sleep makes you more than just tired.
- *Processed Food*: Made with chemicals.
- *Food Sensitivity*: Our immune system can over react to certain foods.
- *Refined Sugar*: But it tastes so good.
- *Animal Fat*: Not all protein is created equal.
- *Hydrogenated Oils*: Too much of a not-so-good thing.
- *Free-radical Damage*: A by-product of the aforementioned behaviors.
- *Obesity*: One more reason to shed some pounds.
- *Excessive Insulin Levels*: Often related to refined sugar intake.
- *Smoking*: No list is complete without it.

How Does Diet Cause Inflammation?

Over and over we hear how the food we consume helps to determine our wellness. Here is another reason to watch what you put into your body and determine if it is worth it. Look at the list of things in the

diagram below that can increase inflammation. Several pertain specifically to types of
foods that are readily found in the typical
modern diet.

Foods containing hydrogenated fats and
refined sugars increase inflammation in the
body. These foods and our bodies' natural
response to them encourage the chronic,
low-grade inflammation that contributes to
degenerative disease. According to study
published in the American Journal of Clinical Nutrition, trans fatty acid
consumption increases inflam-
mation, damages health and has
a strong relationship to heart
disease (Mozafarrian, 2004).

The link between inflammation
and food is so strong that experts
and non-experts alike are creating "anti-inflammatory diets."
Just as there are foods that
stimulate inflammatory responses
in the body, there are foods that
have anti-inflammatory properties
as well.

Adding anti-inflammatory foods
to your diet can reduce inflammation, lower your risk of heart
disease, stroke, cancer, and other
conditions. These foods may also
provide benefits for conditions
such as osteoporosis, age-related
memory loss, and macular degeneration. More about healthful
foods and their benefits later.

My Experience with Food Sensitivity Testing

Last year my husband and I con-
sulted a Functional Medicine doctor
for extensive food sensitivity testing.
The testing showed that my husband
had a moderate gluten sensitivity and
after following a low-gluten eating
plan, he found that a lot of his gastro
intestinal symptoms eased

It became clear to me that there is a
difference between a food allergy that
can have an immediate reaction and
a food sensitivity that might be more
subdued with symptoms of discomfort
building over time. However, they are
both inflammatory reactions.

I am learning that food sensitivity
can go undetected because it may
be masked as digestive problems.
The truth is, the root of the digestive
issue-the indigestion, the gas, the
heartburn, the acid reflux-may be
food sensitivity which can cause
inflammation in the digestive tract.

Sugar and Inflammation

One "food" that perpetuates chronic inflammation is sugar. Refined
sugars, such as white flour, white rice and artificial sweeteners, and

soda (liquid sugar) are big triggers for internal inflammation. Sugars are found in many foods and much of it is hidden. Most people have no idea that sugar comes in many different forms. Here are some of the hidden sugars to look for when reading food labels:

- BROWN RICE SYRUP
- CANE SUGAR
- MALTOSE

- SUCROSE
- MANNITOL
- CORN SYRUP

When blood sugar is high, the body generates more free radicals.

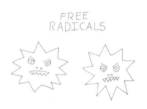

These rogue molecules surge through the body and cause damage to the cells which stimulates the immune response and inflammation in the lining of the blood vessels. The more sugar we put into our bodies, the more free radicals are produced. The more free radicals are produced, the more damage they do to our cells. The more damage sustained by our cells, the more our bodies respond with more inflammation.

Unfortunately, the inflammatory response initiated by the immune system can create barriers in blood vessel walls that make other body processes work less efficiently. A destructive cycle is put into place.

In the development of heart disease, the type of carbohydrates in our diets may be as important as the type of fats we choose, according to Walter Willett, MD, professor of epidemiology and nutrition at the Harvard School of Public Health (HSPH) and author of *Eat, Drink and Be Healthy*. In his book, he explains that the more refined carbohydrates we eat, the more likely we are to be supplying our body with more sugar than it can handle with healthy results (2005).

That point hit home when Willett and a team of HSPH researchers looked at diet and health history data from women who took part in the *Nurses' Health Study*. When researchers distilled the numbers, they found a telling parallel between women eating a diet

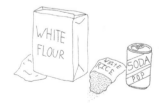

high in refined carbohydrates and those with heart disease. An even more disturbing trend was within the group of women at risk for heart disease. Those who ate the most carbohydrates—including sugars—doubled their risk of heart attack compared to those with diets only moderately high in carbohydrates (Willett, 2005).

When we speak of refined carbohydrates, we are talking about the foods we eat that consist primarily of refined sugars and flour. These include bread products like hamburger buns and donuts; grains like white-flour pasta and sugary cereal; and sugary drinks like soda and sweetened juices. They also include things you may not think about like ketchup, jelly, and sauces.

When the carbohydrates we consume are refined sugar, they cause a spike in blood sugar levels and the body responds with inflammation. High blood sugar can trigger damage to the arterial wall and a whole cascade of events happens as part of the inflammatory response.

Carbohydrates rich in white sugar and flour influence the inflammatory process. We can moderate this process by keeping blood sugar low and stable. In order to do so, we would eat less bread, white potatoes, crackers, chips, pastries, and sweetened drinks. We would eat less refined and processed foods as the refining and processing strips food of its natural fiber. We would avoid fast food and products made with high-fructose corn syrup and other sugars. Instead, we would con- sume whole grains, beans, sweet potatoes, winter squashes and other vegetables and fruits such as berries, cherries, apples, and pears.

Inflammation and Insulin Resistance

There is a real connection between inflammation and the increase of disease in our modern world today. One disease in particular that garners much attention and rightfully so is type 2 diabetes. The obe- sity epidemic that is in full force among young and old feeds directly into the wave of type 2 diabetes sweeping the country and the world. Again, obesity is a major risk factor in the development of pre-diabetes and type 2 diabetes itself.

> ## AVOID REFINED CARBS!
>
> There are plenty of good reasons to avoid the refined carbohydrates that quickly turn into sugar in the body. These carbohydrates deliver excessive and mostly empty calories which instigate inflammation and, therefore, contribute to our degenerative disease epidemic.
>
> In short, our diets greatly impact the amount of inflammation in our bodies. The same list of foods that harm us in other ways, also contributes to an excess of inflammation which has been linked to increased risk for chronic disease.

Less known is the downward spiral of inflammation and insulin resistance that contribute in a dramatic way to diabetes. We've discussed inflammation and its causative role in many chronic and degenerative disease. Now, let's look at the hormone insulin which is central to the type 2 diabetes epidemic.

One eye-opening fact of which I'd like to remind you is that many chronic, degenerative diseases are preventable to some degree or another. Nowhere is that more true than with type 2 diabetes. Lifestyle factors can have a major impact on the development of this disease. Obesity, for instance, is a major contributing factor, and we know that weight is mainly a result of our dietary choices as well as our physical activity level among other lifestyle factors.

The destructive cycle that leads to type 2 diabetes begins with this tiny hormone called insulin. Like other hormones, insulin is a regulatory agent. Its job is to regulate or monitor the amount of sugar in the blood. Insulin is made by the pancreas and is designed to reduce the circulating blood sugar by helping cells take in and use the glucose (sugar). So, insulin's primary job is to control rising blood sugar by driving the transfer of blood glucose from the circulating blood system into other cells.

In order for the body to run at optimal levels, the blood sugar must be maintained within certain parameters. An amazing feature of our body is that we have a mechanism in place to keep the blood sugar at optimal levels. When the level of sugar in the blood is either too high or too low, the body takes steps to "correct" the problem.

To combat too much sugar in the blood, the body secretes more insulin to move more of the glucose or sugar out of the blood and into cells residing within the liver, the muscles, or fat. To deliver glucose into cells, insulin attaches to specific receptor sites on the surface of cells. These sites are called insulin receptors. They receive the glucose from the blood in order for the body to normalize the level of blood sugar.

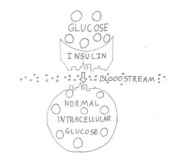

The body never ceases to amaze me. It monitors and compensates for irregularities within. However, when our lifestyles make the irregularities regular, what is the body to do? The body works overtime to try to bring itself back into balance and after a while the "correction system" does not work properly. If we continue to live in a perpetual state of imbalance, the body's innate mechanisms will not work as well.

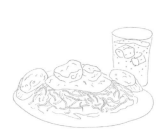

Even the smallest increase in blood sugar levels stimulates the release of insulin into the blood to move the excess glucose (sugar) out of the blood to normalize the levels. That is its job. Unfortunately, we are not usually talking about a small increase in blood sugar levels. Imagine sitting down to a mouth-watering plate of homemade spaghetti with a side or two or white bread and 24 ounces or more of your favorite sugary beverage.

You've sent your body into high alert and insulin spikes. Insulin to the rescue. It enters bloodstream to clean up the mess you've created.

Insulin Resistance and our Diet

The foods we choose to eat dramatically affect the way in which our bodies respond. Carbohydrates that are quickly broken down into their component parts are the same foods that create a spike in blood sugar. When I say "spike," I mean that the blood sugar rises too rapidly. Our body takes the steps described above to counter this "spike."

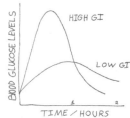

The group of foods that most often contribute to the spiking of blood sugar are certain carbohydrates. These carbohydrates consist of processed foods like potato chips, bagels, foods high in white sugar or some man-made derivative sugar, liquid sugar better known as soda, white carbohydrates such as pasta and potatoes, and fast food.

When you sit down for breakfast with a bowl of processed cereal, half a bagel with jelly, and a tall glass of concentrated orange juice, you've supplied your body with carbohydrates that it quickly breaks down into its component parts. What you may not think about is what these foods are actually made of. SUGAR! That's right. These types of food that break down so quickly and easily provide the body with too much sugar and not enough fiber.

As we've discussed and will continue to discuss, the typical modern diet relies too heavily on processed foods, white carbohydrates, fast food, and sugar. Insulin resistance and pre-diabetes are just some of the results of the devastating way in which our diets wreak havoc on our bodies. In this case, type 2 diabetes has risen to the top of the chronic disease list.

We've already noted the numbers of diabetics worldwide are rising among adults and children. Type 2 diabetes threatens our own health and the health of the rising generations. It is time to understand this epidemic and make real changes in our lives. Let's summarize the steps that can lead us to full blown type 2 diabetes since it looks that many of us are on our way there. It is quite simple and simply devastating.

Stage 1 - "Fast-Carb" Diet

Stage 2 - Insulin Overstimulation

Stage 3 - Insulin Resistance

Stage 4 - Type 2 Diabetes

Stage 1 "Fast-Carb" Diet

The term "fast-carb" refers to carbohydrates that cause the level of sugar in the blood to rise rapidly. These foods spike the blood sugar and stimulate the release of insulin from the pancreas. Simple.

These consist of:

- Processed foods
- Foods high in white sugar
- Liquid sugar such as sodas
- White bread, white rice, white pasta

Stage 2 Insulin Overstimulation

It is common for us to spike our blood sugar many times throughout the day. Just look at what we eat. This continual spiking means insulin is also being continually spiked to keep blood sugar stable.

One of the most serious effects of overstimulation of insulin is the damage that starts to take place in the fine arteries of the body. Elevated blood sugar and the subsequent high insulin levels is a major cause of inflammation of the arteries.

Stage 3 Insulin Resistance

Insulin resistance is the body "resisting" the actions of insulin, therefore, insulin does not work properly. It is not doing its job.

The pancreas responds by producing more insulin. Excess glucose builds up in the bloodstream because insulin cannot work properly, and insulin levels climb. Many people with insulin resistance have high levels of both glucose and insulin circulating in their blood at the same time. This is setting the stage for type 2 diabetes.

Stage 4 Type 2 Diabetes

Here's the clincher. In the beginning stages of insulin resistance the pancreas compensates by producing more insulin to try and regulate blood sugars. Eventually, the pancreas becomes exhausted and no longer compensates. As the cells of the pancreas become exhausted blood sugars start to rise. This is the beginning of type 2 diabetes.

I have witnessed so many people successfully reduce their risk of type 2 diabetes with my program. Here is a success story:

At 54, my doctor first talked about a pre-diabetic result in my annual blood test and I understood that my health was not headed in the right direction.

I started with the five day sugar cleanse and I found the 5-day

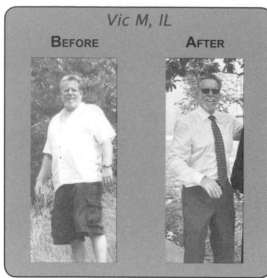

Vic M, IL

BEFORE   AFTER

experience effortless. I liked the taste of the foods I was eating and was never hungry. I began to realize what it meant to truly feel great. I had more energy than I'd experienced in years.

At the end of the 5-days I had lost 8 pounds. I was surprised and thrilled. I continued with the meal replacement shakes for breakfast and lunch each day. I found low-glycemic eating was easy to follow, and the pounds dropped off.

I began to exercise for the first time in my adult life. After four months, my cholesterol, triglycerides, and fasting blood sugar levels were all in the normal range. An added benefit is that my rheumatoid arthritis was also under control and I no longer took pain medication.

In all, I lost 40 pounds in about 5 months time. This corrected a variety of health problems, and I felt boundless energy, allowing

WHAT IS PREDIABETES?

Prediabetes refers to a condition wherein blood glucose levels are higher than they should be but are not yet high enough to render a diagnosis of diabetes. Prediabetes can occur in any stage leading up to type 2 diabetes. When you have prediabetes, you are at increased risk of developing type 2 diabetes.

According to the National Diabetes Information Clearinghouse website, "Studies have shown that most people with prediabetes develop type 2 diabetes within 10 years, unless they lose 5 to 7 percent of their body weight—about 10 to 15 pounds for someone who weighs 200 pounds—by making changes in their diet and level of physical activity. People with prediabetes also are at increased risk of developing cardiovascular disease" (2008).

me to take up running and biking. Four years later, the 40
pounds are still gone, and nobody can believe the older pictures
are really of me. I feel better than I can remember and I can't
imagine my life without the benefit of these changes. I'm convinced I've added years to my life! I owe this to the support of my
wife, Dr. Karen Wolfe, and this Lifestyle program.

- Vic M, IL

Are You at Risk?

The devastating thing about chronic, degenerative disease is that the
consequences of our actions are sometimes years in the future. Our
bodies work so hard to compensate for our lifestyles that we do not
realize or notice the harm we are actually inflicting upon ourselves.

Aside from feeling sluggish or bloated, we hardly notice. And if we
don't stop to think about what our lifestyles are actually doing to us, we
continue our self-destructive habits. Although you may not know it and
possibly have never considered it, it is not unreasonable to wonder if
you are at risk.

Because prediabetes (insulin overstimulation and insulin resistance) is
an internal condition, it often has no noticeable symptoms. As such,
the American Diabetes Association does recommend that adults (45 or
older) have a fasting blood sugar level done every year. Risk factors
include the following (list is from National Diabetes Information Clearinghouse website):

- being physically inactive
- having a parent or sibling with diabetes
- having a family background that is African American,
  Alaska Native, American Indian, Asian American,
  Hispanic/Latino, or Pacific Islander
- giving birth to a baby weighing more than 9 pounds or
  being diagnosed with gestational diabetes-diabetes first
  found during pregnancy
- having high blood pressure-140/90 or above-or being
  treated for high blood pressure
- having an HDL, or "good," cholesterol level below 35 mg/
  dL or a triglyceride level above 250 mg/dL

- having polycystic ovary syndrome, also called PCOS
- having impaired fasting glucose (IFG) or impaired glucose tolerance (IGT) on previous testing
- having a history of cardiovascular disease

The Good News

I realize that the outlook may be bleak. However, there is very good news underlying all of this negative talk. The good news is that insulin resistance, prediabetes, and type 2 diabetes (when caught early) can be reversible. The good news is that you can make a decision today to begin to reverse the trend.

Where do you begin? In the same place we all begin to make a change for our health. Our lifestyle. First and foremost, we must make a change in our diets. We begin one small step at a time. Instead of a diet rich in processed, sugary foods, we recognize the benefit of healthful, whole foods.

What else must we do? Physical activity and weight loss help the body respond better to insulin. By releasing weight and becoming physically active, people with insulin resistance or prediabetes reduce their risk of becoming type 2 diabetic. Physical activity helps muscle cells use blood glucose for energy by making them more sensitive to insulin.

So the good news is that people with insulin resistance or prediabetes can help their body utilize insulin by being physically active, making wise food choices, and reaching and maintaining a healthy weight.

Is Your Lifestyle Killing You?

The fact that our lifestyle plays a major role in our health is irrefutable. We must concede that our habits are contributing to the obesity and chronic illness epidemics. In the next chapter, we will explore eight lifestyle factors that negatively affect our well-being.

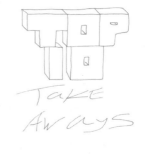

DR. KAREN'S TOP TEN TAKEAWAYS
FROM
THE PRICE WE PAY

1. Excess inflammation may be the highest price we pay for our killer lifestyles.

2. Inflammation plays a significant role in the obesity and chronic disease epidemics.

3. Hidden inflammation can trigger chronic disease.

4. Certain foods can trigger low-grade inflammation that contributes to disease.

5. Refined or processed foods can be big triggers for internal inflammation.

6. Too much sugar leads to too much insulin.

7. The overproduction of insulin leads to inflammation.

8. Insulin resistance, prediabetes, and type 2 diabetes are often related to lifestyle.

9. Different habits today can impact the damage tomorrow.

10. Lifestyle choices influence insulin resistance and prediabetes.

CALL TO ACTION
WHAT YOU CAN DO

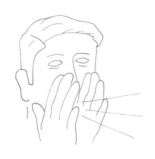

• Remove crackers, chips, pastries, and sweetened drinks from your house.

• Review the illustration that lists foods that increase inflammation and consider reducing or eliminating these foods from your diet.

• Review the illustration that lists foods that decrease inflammation and consider increasing these foods in your diet.

• Determine if you have a sensitivity to a particular food by eliminating it for at least two weeks and see if symptoms such as lethargy, headaches, or bloating subside.

• Avoid fast food and products made with high-fructose

corn syrup.

- Do not eat processed cereal.
- Eat breakfast every morning.
- Eat less bread and white potatoes.
- Eat less refined and processed foods.
- Eat whole grains, beans, sweet potatoes, winter squashes, and other vegetables as well as fruits such as berries, cherries, apples, and pears.
- Exercise daily.
- Check your blood pressure regularly.
- "Know Your Numbers" such as blood glucose, blood pressure, cholesterol.

References

Bakalar, N. (2012, Dec 31). Inflammation byproduct linked to stress. *The New York Times,* Retrieved from http://well.blogs.nytimes.com/2012/12/31/inflammation-byproduct-linked-to-stress-and-depression/

Mozafarrian, D., Pischon, T., Hankinson, S. E., Rafai, N., Joshipura, K., Willett, W. C., & Rimm, E. B. (2004). Dietary intake of trans fatty acids and systematic inflammation in women. *The American Journal of Clinical Nutrition, 79(4),* 606-612. Retrieved from http://ajcn.nutrition.org/content/79/4/606.short

National Institutes of Health (NIH), National Institute of Diabetes and Digestive and Kidney Diseases (NIDDK). (2008). Insulin resistance and prediabetes (09-4893). Retrieved from website: http://diabetes.niddk.nih.gov/dm/pubs/insulinresistance/

Willett, W. (2005). *Eat, drink, and be healthy.* New York: Free Press.

Zappalla, F. R., & Gidding, S. S. (2009). Lipid management in children. *Endocrinology and Metabolism Clinics of North America, 38(1),* 171-183. doi: doi:10.1016/j.ecl.2008.11.006

Chapter 3

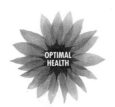

Our
Killer Lifestyles

*We can't solve problems by using the same kind
of thinking we used when we created them.*

\- Albert Einstein

Isn't Einstein brilliant? We have created lifestyles that have led to a global epidemic of obesity, diabetes, and chronic illness. To solve this problem, we have to think differently.

Even in lands of plenty, we are hungry nations. In the United States, in Australia, in Canada, in Japan, in Taiwan, in Hong Kong, and in other developed nations, we hunger for something. Many people are malnourished in these lands of plenty.

Our cells and our bodies are hungry, even starving, for proper nutrition. So often the foods we consume are not real. They are processed with chemicals to improve their shelf life rather than provide meaningful nutrition for our bodies.

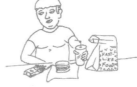

Consequently, these foods are not providing the necessary nutrients our cells need for all the chemical reactions that need to occur for optimal health and basic body functioning. A huge biochemical imbalance is set up.

We spoke about cravings in the first section. One way our bodies signal a nutrient deficiency is through cravings. Cravings can also be the body's signal for an underlying imbalance. They can be important messages meant to signal actions we need to take so that we can get back into balance. When our cells hunger for something, we crave.

Sick and Overweight

We must be honest and understand how we arrived at this place—sick and overweight. The root cause is the change in the way that we live our lives. Although we've advanced in many ways, there are unintended consequences to our modern lifestyle.

Imagine for a moment you are commuting to work. We've all experienced being stuck in traffic when we are already running late. We finally get moving and the distracted driver ahead of us slams on his brakes and we just miss his back bumper.

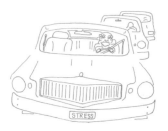

We've all experienced running home from work feeling so tired that making dinner seems an impossible task. Hanging on the refrigerator is the number to the local pizza joint. It's so much easier to pick up the phone and place an order. We've all experienced getting to bed too late and cringing when the alarm goes off too early the next morning. We march off to work to spend long hours indoors. We get up only to use the restroom and maybe visit a colleague two cubicles over. We've all experienced taking a deep breath and choking on the exhaust of the delivery truck as it drives by.

When we want to reward ourselves, we meet friends for dinner and a drink. When we want to be entertained, we go to the movies and sit down for two or three more hours. When we feel sad, disappointed, frustrated, we sit on the couch and watch endless hours of TV while eating potato chips and ice cream.

Does any of this sound familiar?

Obviously, our lifestyle has changed over the course of time. Our modern lifestyle carries with it weighty consequences. The root causes, or the root thought processes that must be addressed are personal, biological, social and economic. Our lifestyle becomes the issue when we look at the levels of obesity and chronic illness we suffer as a nation and a world. Let's look at several lifestyle factors that contribute to the epidemic we are experiencing. What thoughts do we need to address and change? The first factor will come as no surprise, but the magnitude of the problem may.

Lifestyle Factor 1: Poor Quality Food and Food Addiction

Experts once believed that being overweight resulted only from over-eating. This is still the most popularly held belief about obesity. As I write this book, Los Angeles County announced a new public health initiative targeting portion size and caloric intake. It is called *Choose Less. Weigh Less* ("Improving nutrition, increasing").

The campaign is an effort to address the growing obesity rates among Los Angeles residents. Between 1997 and 2011, the rate of obesity nearly doubled (from 13.6 percent to 23.6 percent). The underlying message of the campaign is how much we eat matters ("LA county launches," 2012).

It is true that too much food contributes to weight gain. However, a weight problem is not just about eating too much. It is also about what food we choose to consume. The reason there are more obese and overweight people in the United States than anywhere else in the world is largely due to the amount of processed foods in the typical American diet.

Unfortunately, this reliance on processed food has spread throughout much of the modern world. More and more countries and cities boast super stores where everything from medicine to apples to car tires are sold. This ability to get a product to market and expose it to more and more potential customers is part of our modern way of thinking.

Just about every packaged food product you pick up from the supermarket has been highly processed. When a food is processed, man-made substances and chemicals are added to the food in order to make it look appealing, taste fresher, and last longer. The thinking that got us here now contributes to our problems.

However, the problem doesn't stop there. Most of our commercially available food is highly addictive. Additives that were once used to

preserve the food have multiplied and morphed into substances created to enhance or even create the flavor of the foods we eat. It seems
that no matter how harmful a food or substance may be to the body,
the sensation of pleasure keeps us coming back for more and justifies
its inclusion in the product.

Let's look at two substances that truly affect our bodies in a negative
way: trans fats and refined sugars.

1. Trans Fat

You have heard about trans fat and how horrible it is for you. As if
artificial sugar isn't enough, now we have artificial fat!

Trans fat comes from hydrogenated oils that food manufacturers and
restaurants use to prepare food. The unhealthy fats that end up in our
system from these highly processed industrial oils cause health problems such as obesity, diabetes, cancer, heart attacks, strokes, high
blood pressure, and bad cholesterol levels

Trans fats can keep us overweight. They contribute to hardening of
the arteries which is hard on the heart. They can clog the liver and the
colon which leads to a multitude of digestive disorders and diseases.

2. Refined Sugars

Nearly every packaged food contains sugar, in one form or another.
You will recognize many of the man-made sugars. High-fructose corn
syrup is often an ingredient in foods you may not even realize contains
high amounts of sugar.

Have you checked your ketchup bottle lately? Many products today
contain artificial sweeteners that boast "no calories." We think we are
eating healthy because there are few or no calories in these sugary
snacks. Just because they contain zero calories does not mean they
are healthy. In fact, quite the opposite is true. The chemicals used in
artificial sweeteners can make and keep you overweight.

As we discussed in chapter 1, our brains are extremely sensitive to the
foods that we eat. We've also begun to understand that food can be
addicting just like alcohol and nicotine.

Refined sugar, stripped of its original plant-based context, heavily impacts many physiological systems including our hormonal balance and our gut health. New research is revealing disturbing links between sugar and inflammation. Inflammation, of course, has been implicated as a major factor in a number of diseases, from cancer and diabetes to atherosclerosis and digestive disorders.

Here is a very powerful story from one of my clients who transformed her life by realizing her lifestyle was what needed changing.

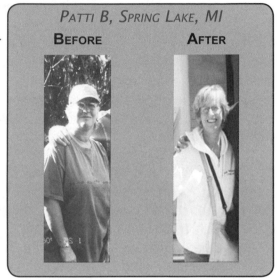

PATTI B, SPRING LAKE, MI
BEFORE   AFTER

I had lost weight many times in my life, but I always gained it back. I tried many diets, and I knew how to count calories and fat--but nothing worked. I blamed it on my age and meno-pause; I was 57. I tried telling myself, "Hey, I'm a grandma and grandmas are overweight."

Around that time, I went to the doctor for my year-ly physical. I was told that my blood pressure was high and I was put on medication. I knew if I didn't do something about it diabetes would be next. I didn't want to go there!

I was desperate. I needed to do something, and I figured I could do anything for 5 days. I decided to do the 5 day cleanse, and it wasn't easy. However, by the 5th day I felt so much better. I had so much more energy and the carb cravings were GONE! My doctor took me off the medication in less than two months.

I continued with Dr. Karen's Lifestyle Plan and added low-glyce-mic meals. I started exercising regularly and the weight started coming off. I lost 10 pounds in the first 3 weeks. I had more energy than I had had in years and all my aches and pains were gone. Over the next 10 months I lost 55 pounds, and I have kept the weight off for 3 years.

- Patti B, Spring Lake, MI

Lifestyle Factor 2: Physical Inactivity

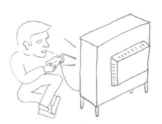

We have become a sedentary people. The ingenuity of people world-wide has contributed to making our lives a life of ease. It is uncommon now that one would spend many hours every day in physical labor. Instead many of us are transported to work each day by car. Where does food come from, according to most of us? The grocery store, of course.

Food that was once grown and harvested by individuals is now mass produced and harvested by machines. Walking used to be necessary to get from one place to another. Today, walking is a form of exercise. Today, the great majority of our population lives in urban areas with little access to outdoor space in which young boys and girls can run and play. Playing is used almost exclusively in connection with video games.

Our Life of Ease Has Become a Threat to our Health.

For years now, we've heard about how important exercise is for good health. We know that without exercise we aren't as healthy as we could be. It comes as no surprise that exercise has numerous benefits. It keeps off excess weight, makes our bones strong, and maintains a healthy heart. What we've never really considered is what not exercising does to our body.

Think about it for a moment. The natural state of the body is move-ment. Our bodies are made for physical activity. Lack of physical movement can cause us to gain weight and develop a variety of obesity-related medical conditions such as high cholesterol, diabetes, and hypertension.

Sometimes we tend to look at exercise as something connected only with weight. Sometimes we think that those who are overweight need exercise more than those who are not. This is to understand only one of the benefits of exercise without recognizing that our bodies were built to move and that the lack of physical exercise harms our body. Here are some ways that the lack of exercise contributes not only to the obesity epidemic but also to the chronic illness epidemic.

1. Lack of Exercise and "Toxic Waist"

We cannot separate exercise and its effect on our weight. Most of us
think of fat as unnecessary storage.   It's a bit
like the storage units so many of us rent to
store our *excess* that won't fit in the house we
live in every day. Well, the idea of fat as just
a storage depot is old science.

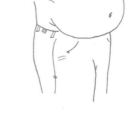

I like to refer to the fat that accumulates
around the waistline as toxic fat. This fat
does not simply wait patiently until we get up
and burn it off. In part, it is toxic because it
actually contributes negatively to our health.
Fat cells, particularly fat cells around the midline, are biologically active and are now considered to be one of the body's endocrine organs
that produce hormones.

Fat cells produce hormones that become part of the total body hormonal communication system. This system sends messages throughout the body to regulate weight, metabolism, and inflammation. That
means that this toxic waist fat puts us at greater risk for cardiovascular
disease. When we exercise, we begin to chip away at this belly fat
that is quite harmful to our health.

2. Lack of Exercise and Constipation

Constipation can be an embarrassing topic to discuss. Despite our
apprehension to discuss matters of colon health, our digestive and
elimination systems have much to tell about our health and well-being.
We will discuss in depth our digestive health later on. At this point,
I want to point out again that physical activity has so much more to
do with our health than weight alone. It is important to note that the
intestinal tract is a long muscular tube. It works much better as a
result of adequate exercise and plentiful water.

Exercise promotes digestion and helps our bodies pass solid waste.
When we don't exercise, the body's digestive process slows and
causes constipation. Constipation then leads to the accumulation of
toxins in the body and inflammation. You are becoming experts on
the topic of inflammation and its role as indicator of ill-health. Aerobic
exercise such as brisk walking, swimming, or cycling gets the blood

flowing to that long muscular tube and the added blood flow helps muscular contractions to help stimulate intestinal function and keep constipation away.

3. Lack of Exercise and Insulin Resistance

We discussed previously that physical activity helps the body respond better to insulin. By being more physically active, people with insulin resistance or prediabetes may avoid developing type 2 diabetes. Remember the healthier the muscle (from physical activity) the more readily muscle cells can accept glucose from insulin.

Physical activity (depending on the type and intensity) can also lower the amount of inflammation our arteries and cells experience, thus improving the rate of success of glucose transfer. To put it simply, physical activity can improve insulin's ability to move glucose into cells and out of the bloodstream. That is a major role of insulin.

Lifestyle Factor 3: Sleep Deprivation

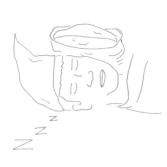

It is common knowledge that adults should get eight hours of sleep each night. For some of you that might seem an impossible task. You work hard every day at work just to come home and see the tasks piling up. Any mother knows that a good night's rest seems a dream more often than a reality. Although we know we need to rest at night and let our bodies and minds relax, we find it difficult to prioritize sleep. Sleep is often the first thing to go when life gets complicated and busy. For some of you, four or five hours a night might seem as good as it's going to get for now.

It is no surprise that a majority of American adults do not get the recommended eight hours of sleep each night. We often relegate sleep to a lesser rung in terms of our overall health. Most of us know that lack of sleep will cause us to be tired and perhaps more susceptible to the common cold, but we rarely consider the effects sleep habits have on our overall health and more specifically here, our weight. They seem to be two unrelated topics when in reality they are connected.

Hungry For Sleep — and Food

Exactly how lack of sleep affects our ability to lose weight has a lot to do with our nightly hormones. Scientists have found that sleep deprivation increases levels of a hunger hormone (ghrelin) and decreases levels of a hormone that makes you feel full (leptin). The effects may lead to overeating and weight gain. The hormones have been called the yin and yang of hunger.

Imagine a traffic light. Green signals "go" just as ghrelin signals hunger. When you have less than eight hours of sleep, the body may produce more ghrelin and signal more hunger. On the other hand, like red signals "stop", leptin signals enough. When you are sleep deprived, your body produces less leptin. More ghrelin and less leptin may equal weight gain for you. Amazingly enough, even our sleep habits can affect our weight and how healthy we truly are.

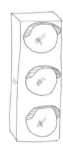

SLEEP AND OBESITY

In April of 2009, a group of sleep researchers convened to discuss studies devoted to understanding the relationship between sleep habits and obesity and type 2 diabetes. Several studies were addressed ranging from how poor sleep affects the body's ability to regulate eating; to sleep deprivation and the body's resistance or sensitivity to insulin; to sleep and the brain and neuroendocrine systems.

Study after study found that sleep contributed significantly to risk factors that lead to obesity and type 2 diabetes. On the ScienceDaily website, a review of the symposium concludes by saying:

The scientists agree that as sleep curtailment becomes more common in industrialized countries it becomes increasingly important to understand how limited or poor quality sleep produces changes that can lead to obesity and diabetes, both epidemic in the developed world. More and more scientists are jumping on board with these lines of investigation, says [one scientist], and there is an increased demand for information on the part of health professionals and members of the general public, many of whom consider themselves sleep deprived (Federation of American, 2009).

Sleep and Inflammation

Our sleep habits can have an additional effect on our health. We've discussed at length the role of inflammation in the disease process. Believe it or not, we need to revisit the idea of inflammation in connection with sleep and the lack thereof. Poor sleep for even a night can lead to the production of damaging inflammatory compounds.

Research has helped us to understand the association between sleep deprivation and increased risk of a wide spectrum of medical conditions including type 2 diabetes and obesity. In our fast-paced, hectic life, we need to stop and recognize the impact a good night's sleep can have and the devastation consistent lack of adequate sleep can have on our health. Sleep is vitally important to maintaining a healthy body.

Lifestyle Factor 4: Digestive Disorders

As surprised as some of you may have been to learn that sleep plays a role in weight and health, you will be more surprised to learn the role of the gut. The gut provides approximately 80% of our immune function. Therefore, good digestive support is absolutely critical to optimal health. I can't stress enough the importance of healthy digestion.

Did you know that your gut serves as your second brain? It even produces more serotonin — known to have a beneficial influence on your mood — than your brain does. It is also home to countless bacteria, both good and bad. These bacteria outnumber the cells in your body, and maintaining the ideal balance of good and bad bacteria forms the foundation for good health — physical, mental, and emotional.

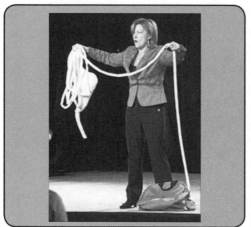

A lot of disease originates in your digestive system. This includes both physical and mental disease. I love to use my model of the gut at my speaking engagements so my audience sees just how amazing and important the digestive system is. One major, often overlooked, contributing factor to weight issues is digestive health. Poor digestive health is often part of the cause of being overweight or obese.

To release weight, you need a healthy digestive system that can absorb important nutrients that enable the system to fight off disease and keep everything running as it should. Virtually all processed foods contain hundreds of additives, toxins, chemicals, growth hormones, trans fats, and sugars. These man-made substances can interfere with our digestive health and can make us fat.

Gut Bacteria and Your Lifestyle

More and more, science is finding that teeny tiny creatures living in your gut are there for a definite purpose. Our large intestine has anywhere from 300 – 500 species of bacteria in it. And we want it that way. Beneficial bacteria, better known as probiotics, are crucial to our health. These microflora can influence our:

- Expression of genes (epigenetics)
- Susceptibility to infection
- Mental health
- Weight

This "good" bacteria gets killed off with excessive use of antibiotics,

---

THE EPIGENETICS FACTOR

HOW LIFESTYLE AND GENETICS INTERACT

Genetics and lifestyle are not as separate as they may appear. We have our own unique set of genetic material that is contained within each cell. Our genome (our hereditary information) comes with a epigenome. Epi means above, so epigenome is above the hereditary information and instructs the DNA to express itself in various ways to create differing expressions.

Epigenetics is the study of how our lifestyle choices can influence gene expression through the epigenome. Although the code itself may not change, the epigenome can. According to genome.gov, "[Y]our epigenome may change based on what you eat and drink, whether you smoke, what medicines you take, what pollutants you encounter and even how quickly your body ages" (National Institutes of Health, 2012).

Genes certainly play a role in obesity and type 2 diabetes (among other illnesses). However, not every person with the gene, or predisposition, develops the condition associated with it. Environmental and lifestyle factors influence whether or not the gene gets switched on to activate the disease process.

---

other medications, toxins, and different foods we eat. This certainly could explain the digestive problems some people have. Your lifestyle can and does influence your gut flora on a daily basis. The flora aids in digestion and absorption of nutrients. These gut bacteria are extremely sensitive to things like sugar and pollution. Sugar can nourish damaging bacteria, yeast, and fungi in your gut, which may actually harm you as much as it impacts insulin resistance.

Damaging bacteria refers to bacteria we don't want in our bodies. These bacteria contribute to our getting the common cold and other inconvenient infections. Other common substances that affect the flora might surprise you: chlorinated water and agricultural chemicals. All of these common exposures can wreak havoc on the makeup of bacteria in your gut.

The Forgotten Fiber

Any discussion of the gut must include a discussion of fiber. Our modern diet often lacks sufficient fiber and a diet rich in fiber not only makes you feel full and aids digestion, but it is also a powerful way to fight disease. According to Mayo Clinic, adequate amounts of fiber in the diet can help to lower the risk of heart disease and diabetes as well as maintain a healthy weight ("Dietary fiber: essential," 2012).

Here are some benefits of fiber, according to Mayo Clinic.

- Helps you maintain a healthy weight because food containing fiber makes you feel fuller for longer.
- Helps to regulate blood sugar levels by slowing down the absorption rate of sugars.
- Helps regulate bowel movements and avoid constipation.
- Helps lower the bad cholesterol levels which helps your heart health ("Dietary fiber: essential," 2012).

Lifestyle Factor 5: Nutritional Deficiencies

In many cases the underlying cause of obesity lies with basic nutritional deficiencies, which can be corrected through dietary changes. These deficiencies are likely caused, in large part, by modern-day lifestyle choices.

More on Vitamin D Deficiency

Two scientists, Gartner and Greer estimated that 70% of America's children are currently deficient in Vitamin D (2003). This is not surprising, given current medical advice. Medical experts often recommend that we avoid the sun to prevent skin cancer. However, the sun is an excellent source of Vitamin D and allows the skin to manufacture Vitamin D directly from cholesterol.

NUTRIENT	EXAMPLES OF DEFICIENCY SOURCES:	SOME ASSOCIATED SYMPTOMS AND DISEASES
VITAMIN D	LOW SUN CLIMATE, IN DOOR LIVING, SUN SCREEN, MINIMAL DAIRY INTAKE	OBESITY, DIABETES, HEART, KIDNEY, MS, OSTEOPOROSIS, RHEUMATOID, CANCER, DEMENTIA
MAGNESIUM	LOW DIETARY INTAKE, DIURETICS, DIABETES, EXCESS SODA INTAKE	MUSCLE CRAMPS, CONSTIPATION, MIGRAINES, HYPERTENSION
IODINE	LOW DIETARY INTAKE, USE OF NON-IODIZED SALT, LACK OF IODINE IN SOIL	FIBROMYALGIA, THYROID DISORDERS, FIBROCYSTIC BREAST DISEASE, THYROID, PROSTATE, BREAST CANCERS

Vitamin D also protects against many types of cancer. In another study, researchers found that Vitamin D deficiency is also associated with an increased risk of high blood pressure and diabetes (Reis et al., 2009).

More on Magnesium Deficiency

Why are so many people deficient in magnesium? There are no single foods that contain huge amounts of magnesium, so there is no magnesium lobby. Look at calcium. The dairy industry constantly tells us that we need to get enough calcium, and we're told right where we can get it: milk and cheese. The same is true with Vitamin C. The orange juice people never let us forget where we can find our daily source of Vitamin C.

Not so with magnesium, so we never really think about it. Another reason that many people are magnesium deficient is that they drink bottled water or softened water. In the old days everyone drank well water or water from streams, both of which contain large amounts of magnesium. Magnesium is removed when water is softened, and most of the bottled waters that are available do not contain large amounts of the nutrient.

You may not have heard much about magnesium, yet magnesium is needed for hundreds of processes in the body. Magnesium plays a role in inflammation, insulin resistance, and subsequent diabetes. In a study published in Diabetes Care, researchers found that magnesium can reduce the risk of developing diabetes (Kim et al., 2010).

Lifestyle Factor 6: Stress

Stress in itself is neither good nor bad. We have a built-in stress-response mechanism where stress hormones make fuel and energy available to help us respond to challenges. However, chronic stress can have a dangerous and even life-threatening effect on the body because it never allows the body to switch off the stress response. Chronic stress can increase your vulnerability to colds, fatigue, and infections.

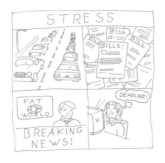

Given the current economic crisis and the high-levels of unemployment in the US and around the world, it is not surprising to note that stress contributes significantly to our health problems. Our stress levels can be influenced by external forces like losing a job or commuting to work in traffic.

Less acknowledged are the internal factors that also contribute to the amount of stress our bodies feel. The following is a list of possible stressors that we may not consider when we think about stress.

- sleep deprivation
- exposure to household chemicals
- diets
- hormonal changes

When we experience stress, our bodies secrete cortisol. One of the main roles of the stress hormone, cortisol, is to help refuel the body after each stress episode. The benefit of knowing about the stress response and how it works is to realize that unhealthful eating and weight gain are not just about willpower. They are also about living a life of unmanaged stress.

Although cortisol is part of the natural bodily response to stress, excess levels of the hormone contribute to the problem of obesity and chronic illness. Excess levels of cortisol can create:

1. Uncontrollable appetite
2. Suppression of our immune system
3. Belly fat gain
4. Resistance to losing weight
5. Sleep disturbances

Research is beginning to show that stress truly affects our health. According to Mayo Clinic, stress can increase our risk for illnesses such as heart disease, digestive problems, depression, and-you guessed it-obesity ("Stress: Constant stress," 2010).

One of my wonderful clients, Dody, shares her story of how caring for her mother created a stress in her life that took her own health on a downward spiral.

My nemesis, for much of my life, was how I felt about my body. Even when I was younger and played racquetball, biked, hiked and swam, I hated how it looked. As menopause hit and the aches and pains increased, so did the underlying hatred. I responded by giving my body sweet things to eat.

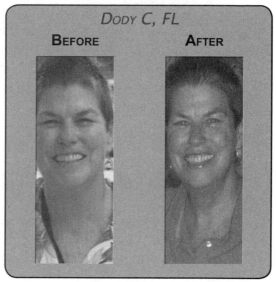

DODY C, FL
BEFORE   AFTER

In 2004, my mom's health failed and my own self-care took a backseat to a 10 hour work day and taking care of her. The pounds followed.

More than a year after my mother's death, I met Dr. Karen at a women's workshop. Her responses to me reached deep into that place where hatred had covered hurt and fear. Her unconditional encouragement to never give up fed my own desire to keep moving forward. My mantra became stay the course. I began The Healthy Lifestyle Solution Program with a bolstered spirit. This program has surpassed 'temporary' for me and has become a major player in supporting a healthier lifestyle.

Swimming is the best exercise for me to support my aging joints and add fresh air to my spirit. My road to restoration has not been a smooth one; there are still potholes, small ones. Dr. Karen's encouraging words reverberate and, once again, I stay the course--size by size!

- Dody C, FL

Lifestyle Factor 7: Environmental Toxins Create "Toxic Fat"

Scientists, environmentalists, politicians, alternative medicine practitioners, and others have been talking about our toxic environment for decades now. Most of us understand that there are dangerous chemicals in the air we breathe, in the water we drink, in the food we eat, and the products we use. Environmental toxins seems inescapable. And they may be, but it is hard to know where to begin to take action.

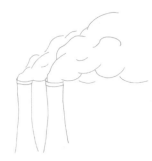

I integrate environmental wellness into my teaching and coaching. Research is revealing surprising health risks posed by our everyday products and habits. Almost overnight, a toxic world has been built around us. Passing on the processed foods in your diet isn't enough; you have to remove toxins from your HOME, too. From household cleaning products to cosmetics and cooking tools, limiting your exposure to household toxins will help reduce hormonal threats.

MAKE YOUR HOME A HEALTHY HOME

As you go through your home and remove products that may not be as safe as you thought, check out your hand soaps. If they are anti-bacterial, read on . . .

In an article in Natural Life magazine, the author summarized information about antibacterial cleaners as follows:

Microbiologist Dr. Stuart Levy of Tufts University told an International Conference on Emerging Infectious Diseases in Atlanta, Georgia in 2000 that strong antibacterial cleaners are needed only when someone in a household is seriously ill or has low immunity. He said that older cleansers such as soap and hot water, alcohol, chlorine bleach and hydrogen peroxide are sufficient for most purposes.

In fact, your use of antibacterial cleaners may be hurting your baby's immune system rather than keeping her healthy. Dr. Levy, who has long been active with the Alliance for the Prudent Use of Antibiotic (APUA), spoke of an Italian study that found that exposure to bacteria is essential for development of an infant's immune system. A baby, he said, must be exposed to germs during its first year in order to develop the antibodies needed to fight infection later in life. (Priesnitz).

I am always interested in helping people to take action to create healthy lifestyles, so I was delighted when Dr. Myron Wentz and Dave Wentz published the book, *The Healthy Home: Simple Truths to Protect Your Family From Hidden Household Dangers*.

I have used this book for book study groups where we have been able to take one chapter at a time and discuss solutions to help minimize toxic exposure in each room of our homes. It is easier to make changes when we have support and encouragement and practical solutions.

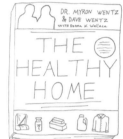

Young mothers attending my book study groups have realized that children's developing brains and bodies (especially their reproductive systems) are extraordinarily vulnerable to toxic chemicals. Children's bodies may not metabolize and excrete toxic chemicals as readily as adults. So it's important for our children's long-term health that we focus on the toxic chemicals they're exposed to, and that we do our best to keep them away when it matters most.

I personally have changed all my cookware in the kitchen, and my personal care products now have no parabens (a common preservative). I have become more aware of chemical exposure in cleaning products and dry cleaning chemicals. As I write this I realize I really have made significant changes for my family as a result of Wentz' book!

Lifestyle Factor 8: Our Environments Support Poor Choices

The best way to illustrate the connection between our social lives and our health is to have you remember a time in which you were determined to change some unhealthy habit for a healthy one. For instance, you may have decided one day to eat less fast food. This is an admirable goal. We all know we should eat less fast food.

The first day, you notice how many fast food restaurants you pass on your way to work or dropping the kids off at school. You begin to notice how many commercials and billboards advertise happiness, friendship, and family togetherness as the actors sit down to a particularly unhealthy meal of fried foods and sugary drinks. The contrast between the vitality of the actors and the reality of the product they represent goes unquestioned most of the time.

Despite the lie these advertisements peddle, they illustrate the relationship the fast food industry plays in our social lives: play dates at the local fast food place, lunch with co-workers at a nearby hamburger place, or family night at the neighborhood pizza joint. Truthfully, it is hard to imagine a life without these common, worldwide companies and their products. They are, in fact, woven into the very fabric of our modern lifestyle.

The obesity epidemic, as well as the chronic disease crisis, may be as much a social disease as a biological or physical one. Our social networks and their ties to dietary habits and other lifestyle habits are telling. Studies are beginning to show a link between our social environment and our health.

In Annual Review of Public Health, while acknowledging there is much research left to do and more to understand, health experts Yen and Syme conclude that studies "suggest that the social environment influences disease pathways" (1999).

What are some of the "social" influences to our health? Let me suggest some. Here is a small list of how I have noticed different "social environments" contributing to the problem of obesity and subsequent chronic disease.

Food Marketing

Media marketing of fast food, junk food, and processed food to children.

- Health claims on food labels
- Schools
- Junk food in schools is often a revenue generating item
- Location of fast food restaurants near schools
- Athletic events

Have you noticed food and soda companies sponsoring the Olympic Games and other sporting events?

DR. KAREN'S TOP TEN TAKEAWAYS
FROM
KILLER LIFESTYLES

1. Most of our commercially available food is highly addictive.

2. Physical activity may help people with prediabetes avoid type 2 diabetes.

3. Belly fat correlates to cardiovascular disease and diabetes.

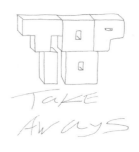

4. Scientists have found that sleep deprivation may lead to overeating and weight gain.

5. Limited or poor quality sleep produces changes that can lead to obesity and diabetes.

6. The gut provides approximately 80% of our immune function and food sensitivities can take a toll on the immune system.

7. In many cases the underlying cause of obesity lies with basic nutritional deficiencies.

8. Excess levels of cortisol contribute to the problem of obesity and chronic illness.

9. Passing on the processed foods in your diet isn't enough; you have to remove toxins from your home, too.

10. Our social environment contributes to our unhealthy lifestyles.

CALL TO ACTION
WHAT YOU CAN DO

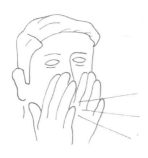

• Eat a diet that includes whole foods rich in fresh vegetables and fruits that provide good nutrients and fiber.

• Replace rice with Quinoa.

• Reduce your TV time.

• Choose a high-quality supplement. Research nutritional supplements with Lyle MacWilliam's book *NutriSearch Comparative Guide to Nutritional Supplements.*

- Optimize your Vitamin D levels by adequate exposure to UV light and regularly monitor your Vitamin D level with a blood test to confirm your levels are within the therapeutic range of 50-70 ng/ml.

- Reduce corn syrup and high-fructose corn syrup which are often ingredients in foods you may not even realize contain high amounts of sugar (such as ketchup).

- Get eight hours of sleep each night.

- Consider a cup of warm chamomile tea before bed. (It is known for its calming properties).

- Increase your fiber intake to 35 grams per day. Good options include psyllium and ground flax seed.

- Stay well hydrated with fresh, pure water.

- Get plenty of exercise daily.

- Wash your hands!

- Read *The Healthy Home* by Dr. Wentz and Dave Wentz.

References

Dietary fiber: essential for a healthy diet. (2012, Nov 17). Retrieved from http://www.mayoclinic.com/health/fiber/NU00033

Federation of American Societies for Experimental Biology (2009, April 24). Evidence Mounts That Short Or Poor Sleep Can Lead To Increased Eating And Risk Of Diabetes. ScienceDaily. Retrieved January 2, 2013, from http://www.sciencedaily.com /releases/2009/04/090421181032.htm

Gartner, L. M., & Greer, F. R. (2003). Prevention of rickets and vitamin D deficiency: New guidelines for vitamin D intake. Pediatrics, 111(4), 908-910. Retrieved from http://pediatrics.aappublications.org/content/111/4/908.full

Improving nutrition, increasing physical activity and reducing obesity in la county. (n.d.). Retrieved from http://www.choosehealthla.com/eat-healthy/portion-control/

La county launches portion control campaign as obesity rates rise. (2012, October 04). Marketwire. Retrieved from http://www.marketwire.com/press-release/LA-County-Launches-Portion-Control-Campaign-as-Obesity-Rates-Rise-1709503.htm

National Institutes of Health (NIH), National Human Genome Research Institute. (2012). Epigenomics (27532724). Retrieved from website: http://www.genome.gov/27532724

Priesnitz, W. (n.d.). The dangers of antibacterial soap. Retrieved from http://www.naturallifemagazine.com/0602/antibacterial_soap.htm

Reis, J. P., von Muhlen, D., Miller III, E. R., Michos, E. D., & Appel, M. J. (2009). Vitamin D status and cardiometabolic risk factors in the united states adolescent population. Pediatrics, 124(3), e371-e379. doi: 10.1542/peds.2009-0213

Stress: Constant stress puts your health at risk. (2010, Sept 11). Retrieved from http://www.mayoclinic.com/health/stress/SR00001

Yen, I. H., & Syme, S. L. (1999). The social environment and health: A discussion of the epidemiologic literature. Annual Review of Public Health, 20, 287-308. doi: 10.1146/annurev.publhealth.20.1.287

Wentz W. (2012). The Healthy Home: Simple Truths to Protect Your Family from Hidden Household Dangers: Vanguard Press; First Trade Paper Edition.

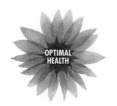

Assess Your

Lifestyle Risk

This assessment is designed to provide you with insight into how lifestyle factors impact your health. Completing this quiz will help you focus on those lifestyle factors that may need attention in your life.

You may choose to go through the final chapter of *Is Your Lifestyle Killing You?* from start to finish, or you may choose to go directly to the lifestyle factor that addresses the area which you wish to focus.

QUIZ
IS YOUR LIFESTYLE PUTTING YOU AT RISK?

Below is a very simple assessment that will help you explore lifestyle factors and health. When you are finished, read the brief explanations at the end.

1. Do you smoke?
- a. No
- b. A few cigarettes a day
- c. 10 or more a day

2. Are you satisfied with the quality and quantity of your sleep?
- a. Yes
- b. Not sure
- c. No

3. Does your breakfast include protein?
- a. Almost always
- b. Sometimes
- c. Never

4. *Your fasting blood sugar is*
>   a. Under 100 mg/dl
>   b. 100 to 125 mg/dl
>   c. 126 mg/dl or higher

5. *You drink two or more glasses of sugary drinks a day (such as fruit juice and soda)*

>   a. Never
>   b. Sometimes
>   c. Always

6. *How much time do you spend each week on a physical activity that makes you sweat?*
>   a. 2 hours or more
>   b. Up to 2 hours
>   c. Zero

7. *You do strength training*
>   a. At least twice a week
>   b. Less than twice a week
>   c. Never

8. *How would you describe the level of stress in your life?*
>   a. Moderate and manageable
>   b. Getting out of control
>   c. Out of control and interfering with your life in a major way

9. *You sit and watch TV*
>   a. Between 0 to 1 hour per day
>   b. 2 hours per day
>   c. 2 + hours a day

10. *How often do you eat every day?*
>   a. Three moderate meals and several small snacks
>   b. Three square meals
>   c. I skip some meals

11. *You sauté vegetables in*
    a. Olive Oil
    b. Vegetable Oil
    c. Butter

12. *You have started to detoxify your home*
    a. Yes
    b. No, but I have a plan
    c. You have no idea where to begin

13. *Do you get constipation*
    a. Never
    b. Sometimes
    c. Often

14. *You spend time with friends that you truly care about*
    a. Often
    b. Sometimes
    c. Rarely

SCORING
Give yourself:

- 3 points for every A answer,

- 2 points for every B answer, and

- 1 point for every C answer.

WHAT DOES YOUR SCORE MEAN?	
Score	**Meaning**
From 23 – 14	Careful! Find a support system and plan some lifestyle changes.
From 31 – 22	Good! Allow this book to guide you to understanding some good steps to take.
From 42 – 32	Great work in practicing good wellness habits.

ASSESS YOUR ANSWERS
The best response to every question is A. Here is why

1. *Stop Smoking* - According to a study published in the *American Journal of Epidemiology*, smoking 16 to 25 cigarettes a day increases your risk for type 2 diabetes to three times that of a non-smoker.

2. *Sleep Well* - Short sleep duration is associated with impaired glucose tolerance and an increased risk of diabetes and lack of sleep is a chronic stress that can increase risk of infection. Also, more than 8 hours of sleep is associated with an increased risk of obesity.

3. *Eat Breakfast* – Most people do not include protein with breakfast. Another common problem I encounter with my clients is the habit of skipping breakfast.

4. *Focus on Fiber* – Foods high in fiber slow the absorption of glucose into the blood stream which helps regulate healthy blood sugar levels.

5. *What's Your Number?* – Schedule a blood sugar test if you are 45 or older or you are overweight or have any of the other risk factors.

6. *Stop Drinking Sugar* – Studies show that people who drink sugary beverages, such as soda and fruit juices, have a higher risk of diabetes even at normal weight.

7. *Sweat for Success* – People who do not exercise increase their risk of type 2 diabetes.

8. *Meet Your Muscles* – Strength training builds muscles. With more muscles, you can improve insulin sensitivity and by so doing, better regulate blood sugar.

9. *Stress Less* – The stress hormone cortisol triggers the release of extra blood sugar because the body thinks you need to flee from danger. It also directs the body to store fat in abdomen which increases your risk for insulin resistance and diabetes.

3A-4

10. *Get Off the Couch* – Exercise keeps muscle cells sensitive to insulin which is the hormone that ushers blood sugar into cells with the result of lowering circulating blood sugar levels.

11. *Eat Regularly* – Eating small meals frequently is better for blood sugar control than a few large meals. Make it convenient to eat a healthy low-glycemic snack, so you won't need to rely on what our convenience culture makes available to you.

12. *Use Good Fats* – Good fats such as flaxseed oil, avocado, and nuts are your preferable fats.

13. *Detox Your Home* – I recommend the book called *The Healthy Home: Simple Truths to Protect Your Family from Hidden Household Dangers* by Dr. Myron Wentz and Dave Wentz. I have found this book to be extremely helpful as I take the steps to detoxify my home.

14. *Gut Matters* – Constipation is a sign of digestion problems. The main cause is dehydration and lack of fiber. Unfortunately, too many of us suffer from some type of digestive problem. Our modern diet often lacks sufficient fiber.

15. *Seek Support* – One of my favorite books entitled *Love and Survival* by Dean Ornish is listed in the RESOURCES SECTION. Here is a quote from that book:

> *I am not aware of any other factor in medicine – not diet, not smoking, not exercise, not stress, not genetics, not drugs, not surgery – that has a greater impact on our quality of life, incidence of illness and premature death from all causes than social connections.*

Chapter 4

The Process to Recovery

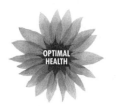

I am a work in progress.
- Violet Yates, Lost & Found

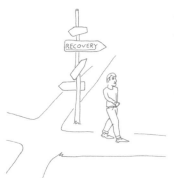

The process to recovery is a process of moving from a lifestyle that enables and promotes disease to a lifestyle that enables and promotes wellness and freedom. Freedom from what, you may ask. Freedom from our own bad habits which have produced in us unhealthy bodies and minds. Our bad habits can sabotage our efforts to live the life we desire—a life full of health and happiness.

Brenda is a person who really understood the transformation needed in her lifestyle and she was delighted to share her story here.

I woke up on the last Tuesday morning in April and said to myself I was either going to accept where I was and know that I would probably die an obese person going into a size 4 X and then 5 X or I would do whatever I had to do to regain my life and my health.

That very day I talked with Dr. Karen and I started the program on Thursday, May 6, 2010.

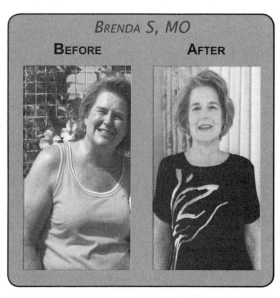

BRENDA S, MO

BEFORE   AFTER

*During the next four months, I shed 45 pounds of fat. I felt unbe-
lievably wonderful. As each day passed, I felt better and better.*

*Knowing what I know now, I understand how much abuse my
body had endured with the unhealthy lifestyle I had accepted and
lived. I had convinced myself that I just couldn't lose weight and
the sabotaging behaviors and destructive lifestyle continued.*

*What I didn't know at the time was that I was insulin resistant and
sugar sensitive. I didn't know the science behind glycemic stress
and carb addiction. Through webinars, education, and support
I learned how to care for my body by incorporating low-glycemic
eating, drinking lots of good water, and supporting my cells with
good supplements. I was being restored mentally and physically.*

- Brenda S, MO

Our lifestyle has to do with the daily lifestyle choices we make regard-
ing the foods we consume, the level of physical activity in which we
engage, our sleep patterns, our digestive wellness, the nutritional deficiencies we may experience, the level of stress we feel and how we
deal with it, the toxins in our environments, and our social networks.

We have discussed extensively the results of our poor lifestyle choices on
our health. Our focus has been on the negative effects of these choices.
Let's now focus on what can happen when we make good choices.

Because our dietary choices impact our health in such a dramatic
way, food is the first step on the road to recovery. However, I make it
a point to teach my clients that this recovery is not a diet. It is exactly
what it sounds like. It is a lifestyle change.

Each of the lifestyle factors mentioned above, and discussed in depth
in Chapter 3, combine to create what I call *The Healthy Lifestyle Solution*. Let's understand, then, that diet is only the beginning. Address-
ing each of the other lifestyle factors is vital to recovering from the
poor choices and habits we've developed. My plan--the plan I used in
my own life and the plan I teach my clients--is a complete action plan.

The Final Piece of the Puzzle - Glycemic Index

In order to fully understand and appreciate *The Healthy Lifestyle
Solution* that will be discussed in the next chapter, we must fill in

another piece of the puzzle. This has been such an important aspect in my work with my clients that I made a special section here to walk you through it.

You may have heard of the glycemic index, but let's explore together the power of low-glycemic choices. I have found this concept to be highly successful in my own life and in the work I do with my clients as I coach them toward their optimal wellness.

My Experience with Glycemic Index

I remember when the United States Department of Agriculture (USDA) food pyramid was created in 1992. The food pyramid was divided into six horizontal sections representing different food groups. The biggest section on the bottom recommended 6-11 servings of a group which included bread, cereal, rice and pasta.

There was a lot of criticism of the original food pyramid. One serious objection I had was the type of carbohydrates shown in the largest section at the bottom of the pyramid. I was pleased to see the USDA roll out its new MyPlate program in 2011.

MyPlate is divided into four slightly different sized quadrants. Fruits and vegetables take up half the space, and grains and protein comprise the other half. The vegetable and grain portions are the largest of the four. This change reflects our new understanding of carbohydrates. So what is it about carbohydrates that contributed to this shift?

All Carbohydrates are NOT Created Equal

We've discussed much about diabetes throughout this book. Let's visit the subject again with a focus on carbohydrates. Years ago, diabetics were encouraged to eat according to what was called dietary exchanges. These simple charts steered diabetic patients away from "simple" carbohydrates and toward "complex" carbohydrates. Carbohydrates were classified as "simple" versus "complex", as you may have guessed, due to their believed effect on blood sugar levels. Unfortunately, these exchanges were not always successful in controlling glucose levels as expected.

You can probably see the problem. The basis of the dietary exchange was that the simple carbohydrates had a more dramatic and immediate effect on blood sugar while a complex carbohydrate released glucose into the bloodstream more slowly.

Remember that the rapid rise in blood glucose levels initiates a response in the body that leads to increased insulin levels. Increased insulin levels may cause inflammation, and inflammation may lead to other complications.

The 'simple' versus 'complex' theory treated each simple carbohydrate the same; it also treated each complex carbohydrate the same. Simple was bad and complex was good. But not all carbs are created equal.

Exploring the Glycemic Index

Professor David Jenkins of Harvard University began to investigate how and why different carbohydrates affected the body in different ways. He studied individual carbohydrates and their specific effect on blood sugar.

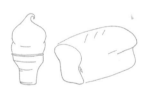

Jenkins and his colleagues found that white bread, a complex carbohydrate, when given in equal amounts, increased blood sugar levels more than ice cream! Nutritionist Johanna Burani noted Jenkins' findings seemed to "fly in the face of the exchange system and the conventional wisdom of the time" (2005).

Other researchers also began studying individual carbohydrates. As more and more carbohydrates were studied, it became clear that the old way of thinking--simple versus complex--did not adequately account for the way in which various carbohydrates affected the level of glucose in the bloodstream.

What Exactly is the Glycemic Index?

The basis of the glycemic index is that each carbohydrate affects the rise in blood glucose differently. The index ranks carbohydrates according to their impact on the level of blood glucose level after the carbohydrate is consumed. The carbohydrate is assigned a number from 0 to 100 that corresponds with its impact on blood sugar levels.

A higher number indicates the carbohydrate causes a more rapid rise in blood sugar level. A lower number corresponds with a slower rise in blood sugar level.

Here is an example of some common carbohydrates and where they fall on the glycemic index. Remember, the lower the number the more slowly the body breaks down the carbohydrate and the more slowly glucose is released into the blood. Releasing glucose into the bloodstream slowly helps avoid the spiking of blood sugar so detrimental to the body. This graph is taken from Burani's article in *DiabetesHealth* (2005).

Food Type/Level	Index
Low: 0 to 55	
Apple	38
Baked beans (canned)	48
Intermediate: 56 to 69	
Raisins	56
Instant oatmeal	66
High: 70 or more	
Cheerios	74
Pretzels	83
Cornflakes	92

Some of these foods and their placement in the glycemic index may surprise you. How many times have you sat down to a "healthy" breakfast of corn flakes?

We often think we are eating healthy foods without realizing that these foods break down in the body too quickly and contribute to increased blood glucose levels, increased insulin levels, and increased inflammation in the arteries.

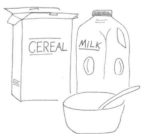

Why is Glycemic Index Important?

I cannot overstate the importance of the glycemic index. You'll recall that the body performs best when blood glucose levels are steady and

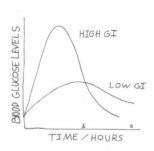

maintained within a certain range. The body responds to an increase or a decrease of blood sugar levels in an effort to restore and maintain the proper balance. It does this by secreting the hormone insulin.

We've discussed insulin extensively. When we follow a low-glycemic lifestyle, we are helping our bodies maintain the proper levels of blood glucose and avoiding the spikes in blood sugar which lead to increased levels of insulin and the consequences that follow: inflammation and insulin resistance.

The relevancy of the glycemic index extends far beyond the scope of diabetes. Learning to eat foods that maintain blood glucose levels within the normal range impact our weight gain or loss, our energy levels, the quality of our sleep, our dependency upon sugar, our ability to concentrate, and our natural ability to feel full.

Introducing Glycemic Load

The glycemic index is only part of the story. How high your blood glucose rises and how long it remains high when you eat a meal containing carbohydrates depends on the quality (Glycemic Index) as well as the *quantity* of the carbohydrate. The glycemic load accounts for the quantity, or the actual grams of carbohydrate per serving, as well as the quality. The following formula is used to find glycemic load.

Glycemic load = (Glycemic Index X Grams of Carbohydrate per serving) ÷ 100

It is possible for a particular carbohydrate to have a high glycemic index but a lower glycemic load. Just as a lower glycemic index is preferable, so too is a lower glycemic load.

It should come as no surprise to learn that most processed, refined carbohydrates have both a high glycemic index and a high glycemic load. On the other hand, fruits and vegetables, legumes and whole grains, tend to have a lower glycemic index as well as a lower glycemic load.

Whenever I research glycemic index I find different scales and different numbers, so my aim here is to simply highlight how to use the formula above and to contrast some popular food items.

Glycemic Load of Popular Food Items				
Food	Serving Size	Grams of Carb. per serving (A)	Glycemic Index (B)	Glycemic Load B x A / 100
Small Apple	120g	16g	39 ± 3	6
Potato	150g	26g	86 ± 6	22
Sweet Potato	150g	32g	70 ± 6	22
Cornflakes	30g	25g	81 ± 3	20
Banana	120g	25g	62 ± 9	16

So you can see that a potato has a much larger impact on blood glucose than a small apple. It is very helpful to use the glycemic load ranking as well as the glycemic index since GI is only part of the story.

Brenda L has a story about how maintaining stable blood sugar levels helped her reclaim her body.

Exercise, health promotion, and disease prevention have been a major focus of my life. As a 35 year fitness professional, a major aspect of my work has been to facilitate various weight management programs, yet the focus has been on behavior change: controlling calories in and calories out. Professionally, I have not supported diets because diets do not work unless one changes an attitude and maintains consistent healthy behaviors.

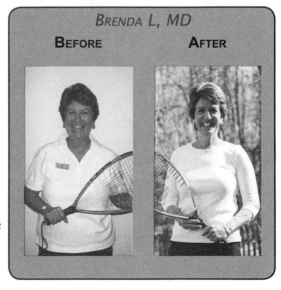

During the past 7-10 years, it had been a struggle for me to figure out how I could lose the extra 15 or so pounds that seemed to be a result of menopause and aging. I had maintained my avid focus on

*daily exercise. My dietary habits were not perfect, but they were
essentially healthy. Yet, I could not seem to get the weight off.*

*In July, 2009, I gave a gift to myself and did Dr. Karen's program
during the week of my birthday and the results were unbelievable.
I was finally able to reclaim my body. Dr. Karen had promised
that certain healthy things would happen and they did. My body
did tell me what it needed; my carb cravings were reduced; and I
felt different.*

Brenda L. from Silver Springs, MD

TOP TEN FAQ's: Glycemic Index and your Health

There are many misconceptions and misunderstandings surrounding
the glycemic index and carbohydrates and how they relate to our
health. The following is a list of common concerns, many of which you
are likely to have.

QUESTION 1 – Does the body need carbohydrates?

The short answer is yes. But let me explain. The body needs carbohydrates because of the glucose they provide for fuel, especially to
the brain. Our brain needs sugar to work. Therefore, the body has a
sophisticated regulatory system designed to keep blood sugars in a
narrow window where the body operates optimally.

As we've discussed, insulin is at the center of the regulatory mechanism controlling blood sugar levels. Let's review the process quickly.
The pancreas releases insulin, and the insulin transports glucose from
the bloodstream to the muscle, liver, and fat cells. Insulin does this by
attaching itself to specific insulin receptor sites on the surface of these
cells and driving sugar into the cells.

At times, the insulin drops blood sugar too low and a counter regulatory hormone called cortisol is secreted to raise the blood sugar level
again. Remember, cortisol stores fat and makes even more glucose.

Let me remind you how dangerous this spiking of blood sugar and
insulin is. High insulin levels and high blood sugar levels both are
pro-inflammatory to the body. That means they both increase free
radicals which sets up an inflammatory response. The inflammation
creates a barrier at the insulin receptor sites (creating insulin resis-

tance) and insulin cannot get glucose into the cell. A chain of metabolic events is triggered that eventually result in elevated blood pressure, cardiovascular disease, obesity, and/or diabetes.

QUESTION 2—What is glycemic load?

The glycemic load takes into account both the quality (the GI) and the amount of carbohydrate consumed in a serving. Glycemic load is calculated as follows:

GL = GI x Net Grams of Carbs per serving divided by 100

As with GI, the lower the glycemic load the less destructive its effect on blood sugar levels. It shows us that the glycemic index is only one aspect we should consider when choosing quality carbohydrates. The glycemic load also helps determine how a food affects our bodies.

QUESTION 3—What is glycemic stress?

Glycemic stress describes the inflammatory cellular response to spiking blood sugar and insulin over time. It is the beginning of insulin resistance and contributes to both diabetes and obesity. Glycemic stress is primarily due to the increased number of free radicals created by elevated blood sugars. We now know that a rapid rise of blood sugar can cause stress to the lining of the small arteries.

QUESTION 4—How is high blood sugar and heart health linked?

Insulin resistance is often called pre-diabetes. Why do we care? Well, one of the most serious side effects of insulin resistance is the damage of the blood vessel system. Elevated blood sugar and insulin in the blood stream is one of the major causes of inflammation in the lining of the arteries.

Most people with insulin resistance do not know it. With no dietary changes, they become increasingly more resistant, which causes insulin levels to continue to rise. If nothing is done to reverse the insulin resistance, metabolic consequences occur. These may include conditions such as elevated blood pressure, changes in blood lipids, cardiovascular changes, and diabetes. Full blown diabetes is held off as long as the pancreas continues to release excessive insulin and keeps blood sugar relatively stable.

QUESTION 5—If I am not diabetic, is the glycemic index important?

Yes, yes, yes. NOW is the time to create healthier choices. It's almost impossible to overstate how serious the effects of diabetes and obesity are. Dr. Christiane Northrup, author of *Women's Bodies, Women's Wisdom*, believes understanding and applying knowledge of the glycemic index is necessary to achieve optimal health (Northrup, 2012).

The important thing to note is that you might feel fine while the process of glycemic stress develops within your body. You may have very few, if any, physical complaints.

QUESTION 6—How is the glycemic index and weight gain related?

This is probably the most commonly asked question. Often we are told weight gain results from a lack of willpower. However, science tells us something different. Insulin is a fat storage hormone. This is important, so I'll repeat myself. Insulin is a fat storage hormone.

When the insulin receptors do not work properly, the body believes there is not enough insulin to get glucose into the cells where it belongs. The body secretes more insulin. The muscle cells quickly become resistant to the insulin, so the glucose from a meal finds its way to the insulin receptors on the fat cells in order to be converted into energy. To make matters worse, the abdominal fat cells, in particular, receive the glucose. The weight happens around the waistline. It is what I call toxic waist or spare tire syndrome.

QUESTION 7 –What role does stress play in the insulin response?

When we feel stressed, our bodies secrete more of the stress hormone cortisol. Cortisol is a fat storage hormone. That certainly doesn't sound good. It also causes the body to produce more glucose which exacerbates the already high blood sugar levels. The blood sugar rises which spurs another surge of insulin. We have too much insulin, so the body secretes cortisol. And the destructive cycle continues.

Dr. Deborah Kern, a health scientist who specializes in mindbody wellness, points out that this creates a triple whammy of inflammation. The excess cortisol creates inflammation as does the excess blood sugar and excess insulin. She teaches ways to stop the endless loop of stress and how to maintain a healthy lifestyle (Kern, 2012).

QUESTION 8 –What role does exercise play in insulin response?

Several studies have provided scientific data revealing how even moderate exercise improves insulin sensitivity. In fact, insulin sensitivity, or the body's ability to transport glucose from the bloodstream to cells, improves in direct proportion to the improvement in physical fitness. Since 80 to 90 percent of our circulating blood glucose is taken up by insulin receptors on muscle cells, the more muscle we have to take up and utilize sugar, the less will go to the fat cells.

QUESTION 9 – What is the role of nutritional supplementation?

In question three, we defined glycemic stress as the inflammatory cellular response that happens over time as we continually cause our blood sugar levels and insulin levels to spike. Eventually, we develop a resistance to insulin and an inflammatory response begins.

This jeopardizes our cellular health. Good cellular nutrition (the word I use for supplementation) enhances our antioxidant defense system, our immune system, and our body's repair system. This gives our body an opportunity to protect our cell walls and blood vessel walls from free radical attacks.

Consuming high quality nutritional supplements that provide all the nutrients to the cell at optimal levels not only helps protect your body, but is essential for lasting vibrant health.

QUESTION 10—Should children follow a low-glycemic diet?

You can never begin too early to instill healthy habits in young people. Too often we allow children to eat foods that are harmful to them because we mistakenly believe they will outgrow them. We console ourselves with the thought that their tastes will change, and one day they will prefer fruits and vegetables to cookies and candy.

In a revealing study published online in Pediatrics, May, Kuklina, and Yoon found a disturbing increase in the number of teenagers with pre-diabetes or diabetes from 2000 to 2008. The numbers increased from 9% to 23% (2012). More and more children are developing a disease that used to be called adult onset diabetes because it was rarely found in children. Unfortunately, that simply isn't the case anymore.

Dr. Christine Wood, a practicing pediatrician and author of the book, *How to Get Kids to Eat Great and Love It*, emphasizes that starting early with habits of eating healthy and staying active is an important part of a parent's job. Every day she sees the reality of poor dietary and other lifestyle choices. Understanding how to encourage low-glycemic choices and limiting processed food choices helps us as well as our children lower our health risks for the future (Wood, 2012).

What is the Solution?

Some of you may be thinking that I've painted a pretty bleak picture here. In reality, we are in a pretty bleak situation. The majority of us have fallen victim to the modern lifestyle of fast food, stressful jobs, inadequate sleep, too little exercise, and emotional imbalance. Is there a light at the end of this tunnel? Is there a silver lining? Of course there is, and the simplicity of it all may surprise you.

The solution I have been working with for over five years now is what I call *The Healthy Lifestyle Solution*. I've called it by other names as well, and I want to share them with you because they too are fitting:

- The Anti-Inflammatory Lifestyle Plan
- The Insulin Sensitivity Lifestyle Plan
- The Releasing Weight Lifestyle Plan
- The Low-Glycemic Lifestyle Plan

The great thing about this plan is that no matter what name I use, the results are the same:

1. Decreased inflammation
2. Improved insulin sensitivity
3. Released fat, especially around the midline
4. Reduced carbohydrate cravings
5. Improved response to exercise
6. Increased energy
7. Enhanced sleep quality

Where Do We Go From Here?

The final chapter of this book will take us down the road to recovery by explaining each positive change *The Healthy Lifestyle Solution* brings. It explains how I have coached many clients to regain their health and create freedom from poor habits through a healthy lifestyle.

I am excited for you to enjoy the freedom of not being addicted to fast food and all the high-glycemic and processed carbohydrates so abundant in our culture. You will enjoy moving your body with pleasurable exercise and reaping the health benefits of removing excess toxins from your life. You will relish the way you feel and have a new energy level along with a sense of well-being. You will be motivated when you begin to shed excess pounds of fat and realize that you are not even trying to lose weight.

This journey down the road to recovery is well worth the effort. A new life is waiting for you!

DR. KAREN'S TOP TEN TAKEAWAYS
FROM
THE PROCESS TO RECOVERY

1. Bad habits sabotage our efforts to live the life we desire.
2. The glycemic index ranks carbohydrate foods based on their impact on blood glucose levels.

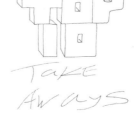

3. Your body performs best when your blood sugar is kept relatively constant.
4. The relevancy of the glycemic index and glycemic load extends far beyond the scope of diabetes.
5. Glucose is the body's energy source.
6. The glycemic load takes into account both the quality (the GI) and the amount of carbohydrates in a serving.
7. High insulin levels and high blood sugar levels are both pro-inflammatory to the body.
8. Glycemic stress describes the inflammatory cellular response to spiking blood sugar and insulin over time.
9. A serious side effect of insulin resistance is damage to the blood vessel system.
10. *The Healthy Lifestyle Solution* is the road to recovery.

CALL TO ACTION
WHAT YOU CAN DO

- Go to glycemicindex.com and look for recipes and meal plans for low-glycemic eating.

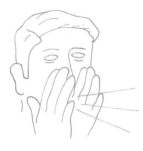

  - Choose complex carbohydrates with a low-glycemic index such as apples, asparagus, beans, broccoli, blackberries, blueberries, cabbage, citrus fruits, green beans, leafy greens, spinach and strawberries.

  - Combine protein and carbohydrates for your meals and snacks as this can lower the GI value of your meal.

  - Never skip breakfast.

- Choose snacks such as olives, nuts, plain popcorn, hummus dip with cut up vegetables, individual low-fat yogurt, or low fat string cheese.

- Choose heart-healthy fats like olive oil, nuts, avocados, seeds, and nut butters.

- Cut back on saturated fats, and remove trans fats completely.

- Choose whole fruit rather than fruit juice.

- Replace instant oatmeal with steel-cut or old-fashioned oats and make sure any cold cereals you use have at least four grams of fiber per serving.

- Choose whole rather than refined grains.

- Aim for vegetables to take up 60% of your plate, protein 25%, and 15% high fiber grain.

- Look for cookbooks that focus on low-glycemic eating.

- Tell your friends who have children about the book *How to Get Kids to Eat Great and Love It*, by Dr. Christine Wood.

- Have your fasting blood sugar level taken and aim for it being under 100.

REFERENCES

Burani, J. (2005, March 1). The glycemic index—a little bit of history. DiabetesHealth, Retrieved from http://www.diabeteshealth.com/ read/2005/03/01/4238/the-glycemic-indexa-little-bit-of-history/

Kern, D. (2012, Aug). Interview by K Wolfe [Personal Interview]. Glycemic index made easy, Salt Lake City.

May, A. L., Kuklina, E. V., & Yoon, P. W. (2012). Prevalence Of Cardiovascular Disease Risk Factors Among US Adolescents, 1999□2008. Pediatrics, doi: 10.1542/peds.2011-1082

Northrup, C. (2012, Aug). Interview by K Wolfe [Personal Interview]. Glycemic index made easy, Salt Lake City.

Wood, C. (2012, Aug). Interview by K Wolfe [Personal Interview]. Glycemic index made easy, Salt Lake City.

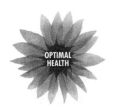

OPTIMAL
HEALTH

Chapter 5

The Healthy
Lifestyle Solution

*I believe most major illness in developed
countries is directly related to lifestyle.
Therefore, I can think of no better medicine
than that of a change in lifestyle.*

- Dr. Karen Wolfe

Beginning Anew

The beginning of a journey brings excitement and a little bit of fear. We are often excited about what the future might hold but fearful of the unknown. The journey to better health is no different. Looking into the future and seeing a new you--free of the extra weight, free of the ill health, free of the disappointment--can be exhilarating and motivational. But fear of the changes and our past failures may cause us to hesitate.

Set aside your fear, your hesitation, your doubt. I invite you to learn about *The Healthy Lifestyle Solution* and to take this journey with me. The success I've seen in my own life and the lives of my clients is undeniable. The plan can and does work in bringing about a lifestyle change that produces in you habits that promote health and wellness. You can take this journey to a better place: happiness. Witness what it has done for Margaret of Chicago:

I never believed I'd lose even a pound unless I became seriously ill. I thought something was wrong with the way my brain was wired because I never received a signal that I was full. After eating a meal, I still wanted to eat another meal. My appetite was intensely strong. I felt as if there were a hungry animal living in my stomach.

When I got on the scale and hit my highest weight ever, I laughed. I had cried in the past, but this time I laughed because I knew the jig was up; I needed to try something. After working with Dr. Karen for five days, a really weird thing happened to me. For the first time, I didn't feel hungry. As I applied what I learned from Dr. Karen's Sugar Busters webinars and support calls, my body calmed down and no longer cried out for food. I had actually given up sugar in 1989. What I didn't realize was the fast carbs in my diet had the same impact on my body as eating sugar, and they were making me hungry.

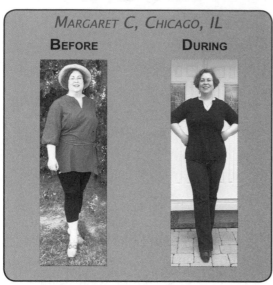

MARGARET C, CHICAGO, IL

BEFORE   DURING

I had always suspected that there was some sort of "trick" to losing weight--a pill or a medical procedure. Turns out there is a trick, but it's not a pill or a procedure at all. It is this: if you don't spike your insulin, your body will release fat.

As I lost weight, people congratulated me and would say things like "I know it's really hard." The funny thing-it actually wasn't hard; it was surprisingly easy. I'm sorry for people who struggle so much because it's not that hard.

Another strange thing happened as I made better choices. I actually felt good. I never knew I didn't feel good, until I actually felt good. At the end of the 5 days, I had released 4lbs. Not bad for someone who thought she'd never lose even a pound. So far, I've lost 37 pounds and am back to my "wedding weight." I still have farther to go to reach my goal, but I'm creating health from within through leading a Low-Glycemic Lifestyle.

I'm so glad I was wrong. I didn't lose weight by becoming seriously ill; I lost it by becoming seriously healthy!

- Margaret C, NW Chicago suburbs, IL

The Healthy Lifestyle Solution 1: The Food Plan, Food as Medicine

Let me remind you that we can consider food a drug. A vital step to improving our lifestyles is proper use of this drug. Food can produce negative effects in our bodies such as spiking blood sugar levels, increasing destructive inflammation, contributing to biochemical imbalance, and creating harmful cravings and addictions.

FOUR REASONS DIETS FAIL

Traditionally, we've believed that weight loss and weight gain were purely a matter of personal will power or the lack thereof. Now you know that weight depends upon much more. Our brains interact with our lifestyle choices to a much higher degree than previously understood. Diets, too, fail for more complicated reasons than lack of willpower. Let's explore four of those reasons:

REASON # 1 – SHORT-TERM MINDSET

Short term restrictive diets encourage you to turn your life inside out for two weeks or so. Yet once those two weeks are over and you return to your old habits, guess what? Your body returns to its former state as well.

REASON # 2 – CALORIC RESTRICTION CAN RESTRICT THE METABOLISM

If you are starving yourself, you're slowing your metabolism and actually burning calories at a far less effective rate than you could and should. You might also be setting yourself up for bingeing because starving people seek out food. When you restrict calories below the basic amount of energy or calories needed to run your basic metabolism for the day, your body will refuse to give up its hold on the fat that you are trying so hard to get rid of. For the average person, your resting daily caloric need is about ten times your weight in pounds. So if you weigh 150 pounds, your resting metabolic need is 1500 calories. This is how many calories your body would need if it does not expend any energy.

REASON # 3 – CALORIE-RESTRICTING OR "CRASH" DIETING STRESS

Stress causes the body to release the hormone cortisol, which fuels the blood with energy in the form of sugar, enabling us to flee from potential dangers. Over time, high stress levels lead to chronically elevated cortisol levels that can cause increased appetite and weight gain.

REASON #4 – DIETING WITHOUT EXERCISE CAN DECREASE YOUR MUSCLE.

Diets also tend to pay too little attention to supporting muscle mass during periods of caloric restriction and so most people who go on a diet lose metabolically active muscle. This is important for more than just aesthetic reasons. When you lose muscle, your basal metabolic rate drops, and you don't burn as many calories. Muscle cells burn seventy times more calories than fat cells. Therefore, yo-yo dieting makes you lose a big part of your metabolic engine.

The Food Plan provides a way to select and prepare foods based on scientific knowledge of how they can help the body maintain optimal health. Along with decreasing inflammation, this food plan provides steady energy, balanced biochemistry, and ample vitamins, minerals, essential fatty acids, dietary fiber, and protective phytonutrients.

Recognizing Sugar Sensitivity

As stated previously, sugar has drug-like properties and can be as addictive to some as cocaine. I have witnessed the power of sugar addiction in my own life and in the lives of hundreds of my clients.

Fast carbohydrates such as those refined, processed foods with a high glycemic index are digested quickly, and they raise blood sugar quickly. This rise in blood sugar produces short-term energy, clarity, and focus. Unfortunately, blood sugar drops as quickly as it rises, leaving you tired, restless, confused, and more irritable than usual.

Slow carbohydrates such as fruits, vegetables, and whole grains, are digested more slowly and provide a slow and steady rise in blood sugar. These slow carbohydrates may not provide the "high" that fast carbs do, but they also don't set you up for the crash that inevitably follows. The slow, steady rise in blood sugar they initiate makes them a much better choice for sustained energy.

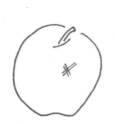

I would like to point out something important here. Fast carbohydrates do not affect all people equally. Some people are more sugar sensitive than others, just as some people are more predisposed to develop an addiction to alcohol. Some people can eat one cookie without wanting another. For others, eating just one cookie seems an impossibility, and eating one cookie leaves them with an overwhelming desire to eat another. One feels so unsatisfying. These people, and I am one of them, are plagued with a sugar craving for the rest of the day.

In her book, *Potatoes not Prozac*, Dr. Kathleen DesMaisons provides a questionnaire to discover whether or not you are sugar sensitive. Check each of the following statements that apply to you:

____ I really like sweet foods.

____ I eat a lot of sweets.

____ I am very fond of bread, cereal, popcorn, or pasta.

____ I now have or have had a problem with alcohol or drugs.

____ I have a parent(s) who is(are) alcoholic.

____ I have a parent(s) who is(are) especially fond of sugar.

____ I am overweight and don't seem to be able to easily lose the extra pounds.

____ I continue to be depressed no matter what I do.

____ I often find myself overreacting to stress.

____ I have a history of anger that at times surprises me.

(This questionnaire reprinted with permission from *Potatoes not Prozac* by Kathleen DesMaisons)

In the questionnaire, the more statements you answered with a "yes", the more likely you are to be sugar sensitive. Being sugar sensitive means that sugar is not simply an energy source for you. It is an addictive substance and you must be extra careful when choosing foods.

You must be ever vigilant, remembering that even though eating simple sugars can temporarily boost your energy level, they ultimately cause your blood sugar to crash. This is true for both sugar-sensitive and non-sugar-sensitive people. However, sugar-sensitive people are compelled to seek more and more sugar, while non-sugar-sensitive people may opt for other food choices.

Dr. Karen's Top Ten Guidelines to The Healthy Lifestyle Solution 1: The Food Plan

Remember that this is a lifestyle change and not a diet. The food plan is simply that: a plan to use food properly. Our relationship with food provides the foundation for *The Healthy Lifestyle Solution* because we can make the greatest impact on our health through the foods we choose.

Solution 1, Tip 1: Consider jump starting your food plan.

Whether we are sugar sensitive or not, most of us have developed unhealthy habits in our dietary choices. Changing our food habits and our relationship to food is not an easy thing to do. Food choices are usually the beginning and the end of our attempts to change.

For this reason, I ask my clients to begin with the 5-day sugar cleanse I have listed in the back of this book. A sugar cleanse serves two purposes.

First, it initiates a thought process and understanding that the body needs a break from the inflammatory foods to which it has become accustomed. It prepares my clients for the predictable physiological stages they will pass through as they change their eating habits. More importantly, it demonstrates that there is a light at the end of the tunnel. Going off of sugars and unhealthful foods doesn't have to be too difficult from a physical standpoint, but it can be very difficult from an emotional standpoint.

The second purpose of the sugar cleanse is much more straightforward. It is actually to cleanse the body. When the majority of the foods we consume contribute to our problems, there comes a point at which we must clear out the old ways and begin anew. The cleanse offers us the opportunity to discontinue our old ways of eating and reset our body's expectations.

Solution 1, Tip 2: Eat protein and "whole" carbohydrates with every meal.

Combining a lean protein with a "whole" carbohydrate can help provide the nutrients your body needs throughout the day as well as help you feel more satisfied. Adding protein to your meals can actually cause you to feel fuller for longer. You already know that fast carbohydrates are too quickly broken down by the body leaving us feeling like we need something more. Slow carbohydrates, which take the body longer to break down, have the opposite effect. Like protein, they help us feel more satisfied. It is really quite amazing how your body responds to nutritious and wholesome food.

Solution 1, Tip 3: Eat every 3-4 hours to keep your blood sugar and insulin levels balanced.

When we discussed blood sugar levels and insulin, we learned that the body wants to maintain the blood sugar within certain parameters. When the blood sugar level is too high or too low, our bodies respond to stabilize blood sugar. We can aid our bodies in this maintenance process by eating every three to four hours to ensure we supply the body with fuel. Often we go long periods of time without eating which causes our blood sugar level to drop. When that level drops too low, our bodies are in a panic to get us to eat. Typically, the meal or snack that follows contains too much sugar and we begin the spiking we really need to avoid.

Solution 1, Tip 4: Eat small snacks with protein – such as a handful of nuts.

Often we feel hungry between meals. Snacking and snack foods can contribute overwhelmingly to our sugar intake. Controlling our snacking is a must. Choose snacks that contain protein and fiber. Check out the call out box for my top ten low-glycemic snacks.

DR. KAREN'S TOP TEN LOW-GLYCEMIC SNACKS

Keep healthy snacks handy! Scheduled snacking is a smart strategy for maintaining stable blood glucose and achieving your weight goal. Snacks help you stay motivated by avoiding hunger, which is what often leads us to abandoning our program. Here are my Top 10 Low-glycemic Snacks:

1. *Yogurt*: Buy low-fat or nonfat, no-sugar added. I love plain Greek yogurt. Yogurts with "live cultures" are healthiest. If you are sensitive to dairy, try a soy yogurt.
2. *Nuts*: An ideal combination of unsaturated fat, protein and carbs. Nuts are portable and nutritious. Buy raw, unsalted nuts or peanuts in the shell; average size is a "handful," about 200 calories, depending on the variety.
3. *Hummus*: Two tablespoons of hummus with cut-up crunchy veggies.
4. *A Hard Boiled Egg*: A perfectly balanced snack.
5. *Peanut Butter and Celery*: One or two celery stalks and 1 tablespoon of peanut butter
6. *Fruit*: Whole fruit including berries, melon, apples, oranges and grapefruit have the most fiber and fewest grams of carbohydrates per serving. Eat along with some nonfat yogurt, low-fat cheese, or a handful of nuts.
7. *Spaghetti Squash*: Baked spaghetti squash topped with vegetables makes a great snack.
8. *Edamame*: One and a half cups of edamame make a great snack.
9. *Eggplant*: I love to saute eggplant in a splash of olive oil.
10. *Low-glycemic Snack Bar*: I always have a healthy snack bar available that has good protein, healthy fats, and low-glycemic carbohydrates to hold my hunger and keep my energy.

When you lose muscle, your basal metabolic rate drops, and you don't burn as many calories. Muscle cells burn seventy times more calories than fat cells. Therefore, yo-yo dieting makes you lose a big part of your metabolic engine.

Solution 1, Tip 5: Beware of night time eating.

Nighttime eating poses a problem for many of us. We tend to want to eat at night when our bodies really need to rest. I recommend to my clients that they eat their last meal two to three hours before bedtime. However, it is not good to go to bed too hungry. Here are a few guidelines I recommend for nighttime eating:

- Don't eat too big a meal too close to bedtime.
- Beware of snacking on comfort foods at night when you relax. These are often loaded with calories.
- Be careful of caffeine as it can stimulate the nervous system and may disrupt sleeping.

The digestive system needs a break just as the rest of the body does. Eating too close to bedtime forces the body to continue working and may cause sleep disturbance.

Solution 1, Tip 6: Always eat breakfast.

One of the most common problems I encounter with my clients is the habit of skipping breakfast. Many of them tell me they skip breakfast and never feel hungry throughout the morning. It is actually more of a problem than you might think.

When you don't eat for eight to ten hours, your body thinks you are moving towards starvation mode; it begins to hold onto fat. Your body is concerned with keeping you alive, not with your weight. Another problem is the inevitable wall you hit mid-morning. At that point, you feel so hungry you eat anything in sight. That anything usually turns out to be some sugary snack.

You need to protect your body by supplying it with the nutrients it needs to fuel your morning. The advice I give to my clients is to eat within an hour of waking up, and to make sure breakfast is hearty. Eat breakfast with protein and a complex carbohydrate each morning.

If you are still convinced you cannot stomach the idea of breakfast, make a protein shake and sip on it slowly throughout the morning.

Solution 1, Tip 7: Always have low-glycemic snacks available.

Sometimes convenience wins even for those with the best intentions. If you are hungry, you are likely to eat whatever is on hand. When you are at work or just around town, what is available is often convenient foods such as cookies, potato chips, candy bars, and soda.

Being serious about changing your lifestyle means being serious about making the right food available at the right time. Here is a list of my favorite low-glycemic vegetables that you can enjoy and have on hand.

- Jicama slices
- Cherry Tomatoes
- Red Bell Peppers
- Cucumber Slices
- Baby Carrots

Make it convenient to eat a healthy low-glycemic snack, so you won't need to rely on what our convenience culture makes available to you.

Solution 1, Tip 8: Focus on low-glycemic foods and make slow-burning vegetables the foundation of your meal.

If you were raised as I was, the starchy portion of your meal covered most of your plate. The token vegetable covered much less. When I went back for seconds, it was almost always a second serving of the rice or pasta rather than a second serving of carrots or spinach. When my plate did consist mostly of vegetables, I felt like something was missing.

It's time to change our minds about vegetables. They truly are the building block for wholesome, healthful meals. They will begin to form the foundation of your eating habits.

Solution 1, Tip 9: Focus on anti-inflammatory foods – wild caught fish, purple and red berries, dark green leafy vegetables.

Remember that inflammation contributes to chronic, degenerative disease. Anything we can do to curtail the negative effects of too much inflammation is well worth it. Certain foods have been shown to have anti-inflammatory properties. Implementing these foods into your diet can moderate the effects of inflammation.

Fruits and vegetables are considered anti-inflammatory foods. We should be incorporating at least five servings per day of green, leafy vegetables and whole fruits. These foods provide vitamins, minerals, antioxidants, and fiber.

Solution 1, Tip 10: Keep a food/feeling journal.

Much of what we feel through our bodies goes unnoticed. We are often so distracted by our environment that we do not hear what our bodies can teach us. Our bodies are, in fact, talking to us. A food or feeling journal can help us document what we are feeling with regards to our food and its effect on us. Our bodies can give us clues and symptoms that hint at the bigger picture. These clues may not be in words, but the body speaks in a consistent and predictable way. Our job is to learn its language. A food/feeling journal can help us become more aware of ourselves. See a sample food/feeling journal below.

Time of day	Food item eaten	Food item desired	How you felt prior to eating	How you felt after eating
_____	_____	_____	_____	_____
_____	_____	_____	_____	_____
_____	_____	_____	_____	_____

Even though emotional eating is not the focus of this book, our eating habits are often tied to our emotions. One of my favorite quotes comes from Gary Zukav in his book *The Heart of the Soul*. "Your emotions are your best friends. They do not leave you. They continually bring to your attention what you need to know. They are the force field of your soul." That statement is so true. Emotions can tell us so many things about ourselves. The topic of emotions and how they are connected with our eating patterns is enlightening and important. If you'd like to learn more about emotional eating please see my book, co-authored by Dr. Deborah Kern, *Create the Body your Soul Desires*.

The Healthy Lifestyle Solution 2: Restore Physical Activity

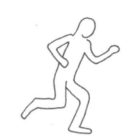

The human body is meant for movement, but movement has been engineered out of our lives. Just think about it. One hundred years ago, normal daily activities such as preparing meals or washing clothes required an enormous amount of physical activity. Today we simply open packages, push buttons, and voila! Dinner is ready! In addition, many of us are glued to chairs in front of computer screens. Forgetting to get up and move can create countless physical maladies. Modern-day life makes it essential to purposely find ways to move our bodies.

Getting and staying fit can be a challenge. For many people, it's hard just to get up off the couch. So what's the secret of people who have managed to make exercise a way of life? Below I reveal my ten top tips for making exercise a way of life and what I have learned about getting the most from my workout routine.

As a reminder, physical activity can help improve insulin sensitivity. When our bodies use insulin more effectively, we are better able to maintain proper blood sugar levels. Physical activity can help lessen inflammation in the body (Ford, 2002).

Dr. Karen's Top Ten Guidelines to The Healthy Lifestyle Solution 2 : Restore Physical Activity

Solution 2, Tip 1: See your doctor before you start any exercise program.

As is true with any exercise program, you need to get a full physical to make sure everything's in working order. Once your doctor has cleared you for physical activity, you could find a personal trainer in your neighborhood and make an appointment with him or her for a consultation. Most trainers will give you a free consultation and help you figure out what your fitness level is, your body fat and measurements, and the right way to start a program.

Solution 2, Tip 2: Maximize the benefit of your exercise routine.

Since so many of us have so little "extra" time to exercise, we must get the most out of the minutes we have! So, regardless of your preferred exercise routine, there are three aspects to include for optimal benefit.

1. *Build muscle* with strength training. Strength training involves resistance to tone and strengthen muscles. Even moderate strength training can build muscle and improve insulin sensitivity. You don't even need equipment, you can use your own bodyweight as resistance by doing push ups, mountain climbers, or pull-ups. Some of the benefits of strength training include:

   - Improved glucose control
   - Improved sleep quality
   - Toned and strengthened muscle

2. *Rev it up* with interval training. Interval training is when you alternate bursts of intense activity with intervals of lighter activity. The pattern is repeated during the workout. For example, you might alternate leisurely walking with periods of faster walking. Whether you exercise regularly or are new to it, here are some of the benefits of interval training:

   - Burns calories faster
   - Adds variety to your routine and prevents boredom
   - Does not require special equipment

3. *Aerobic exercise* is physical activity that causes oxygen to circulate through the blood and breathing rate to increase. A good indicator that you are doing aerobic exercise is that you can carry on a conversation while exercising. (If you are gasping for air while talking, you are probably working anaerobically and are more likely to experience muscle soreness after exercise). Benefits of aerobic exercise include:

   - Improves blood circulation and heart health
   - Improves mood and energy
   - Burns body fat
   - Improves lung function

Solution 2, Tip 3: Set realistic goals.

We have a sad tendency to compare ourselves to others. It is not helpful to expect to do what you see someone else in the gym doing. Be honest with yourself about your physical fitness. Start at a level that is sustainable.

Set goals for yourself that you can actually attain. If you need to begin with a 20 minute walk around the block three times a week, that is where you begin. Do what you can and then build from there.

Solution 2, Tip 4: Use the buddy system.

The buddy system is a tried and true principle. When we have someone to encourage us or whom we encourage, we tend to stay more committed. Have you noticed that you are more willing to follow through on your good intentions if someone else is counting on you?

If you are a person who needs encouragement and a little extra motivation (and most of us are), find a friend, family member, or neighbor who can be your exercise buddy.

Solution 2, Tip 5: Choose activities you like.

We all have different strengths and challenges, different likes and dislikes. When choosing an exercise routine to incorporate into *The Healthy Lifestyle Solution*, be sure to choose some form of exercise that you will enjoy. Enjoying your exercise routine will help you stay more committed to it.

If you enjoy swimming, swim. If you enjoy dancing, you could try a dance class. If you enjoy martial arts, find a routine that is based on a form of aerobic martial arts. There is no shortage of exercise options. Find your place in the world of the physically active.

DR. KAREN'S FAVORITE EXERCISE EQUIPMENT

- Comfortable Walking and/or Running Shoes
- Pedometer
- Water Bottle
- Fit Ball
- Comfortable Work Out Gear
- Resistance Bands
- Heart Rate Monitor
- Jump Rope
- Weighted Ball
- Dumbbells

Solution 2, Tip 6: Try a pedometer.

Do you know how many steps you take in a day? If you are keeping track and trying to walk more, chances are you will take more steps tomorrow than you did today. Step-counters are cheap and easy to use. Best of all, they help you keep track of how active you are. Build up to 10,000 steps a day—or more.

Solution 2, Tip 7: Take the stairs.

A telling symbol of just where we are in our modern-day society is the moving sidewalk. We stand on it and it moves us forward so we don't have to. Don't fall victim to its ease. Walk for yourself, and use the stairs instead of elevators and escalators whenever possible.

Solution 2, Tip 8: Plan exercise into your day.

I'm sure you've heard the adage, "Fail to plan and you plan to fail." I think it is especially true of exercise. If you don't set aside a specific time in your schedule to exercise, it isn't likely to happen. Schedule your day and include time for exercise. Put it in your planner and check it off your list every night. I have my boot camp scheduled in my calendar as an appointment every morning and I schedule other morning appointments around it.

Solution 2, Tip 9: Reward yourself.

This might be my favorite suggestion. When you've accomplished a goal relative to improving your physical well being, give yourself a reward. Maybe you'd be motivated by a relaxing massage or a new set of workout clothes. Have the reward be related to your continued success and involvement with physical activity. My favorite reward to myself is a massage or facial.

Solution 2, Tip 10: Be prepared.

Prepare for your workout the night before by packing your gym bag. Or, if you work out at home, lay out your workout clothes. When you get home after a long day at work, you're ready to go. Personally, I prefer to workout in the morning and begin my day with exercise. I find there are too many distractions as the day progresses.

Does The Thought of Physical Activity Turn You Off?

I know that not everyone who reads this book will be thrilled about the idea of making regular physical activity a part of everyday life. Many of you, like many of my clients, will find this factor to be the most challenging.

Perhaps the thought of physical activity is not on your "must do list" or you might have tried and failed many times. The important thing is to take small steps toward integrating physical activity into your day. We all started somewhere. I have worked with so many clients who found this lifestyle factor to be the most challenging, but they have worked through it and now reap the benefits.

Walking Workout #1
(by fitness Expert Kathy Kaehler)
30-Minutes - Firm Butt & Calorie Burn

You don't always need to speed up or find some hills to blast more fat. Instead, exaggerating your stride length forces your butt and quads to work harder. Alternate one minute of a moderate walk and then one minute of exaggerated strides or lunges to rev up your engine and blast off the calories.

30-Minutes -Firm Butt & Calorie Burn	
Minutes	**Workout Plan**
0:00-5:00	Walk at a moderate pace to warm up.
5:00-6:00	Do one minute of gentle stretching for the lower body.
6:00-9:00	Power surge for one minute, taking the exaggerated strides 6-12 inches longer than your normal stride. Keep a tall posture, looking forward. Alternate between fast pace and normal pace.
9:00-14:00	Power surge for one minute of walking lunges. Lunge forward with your right leg, bending the knees at a 90 degree angle, then rise only slightly to bring your left leg forward into a lunge. Stay low to keep the tension on the thighs. Alternate between one minute of lunge walking and normal pace walking.
14:00-19:00	Return to the one minute of exaggerated strides and one minute of normal pace walking.
19:00-23:00	Repeat walking lunges and normal pace walking for one minute each.
23:00-30:00	Repeat exaggerated strides and normal pace walking and end with a cool down stride to end your walk.

Walking Workout # 2
(by fitness expert Kathy Kaehler)

To double your calorie burn try this blast of energy in your walk. Exchange five-minute chunks of your regular walk with these gradual walk-to-run intervals. In 20 minutes you will torch calories, sweat will drop and you will be energized for hours.

The 20 or 40-Minute Fat Melt	
Minutes	**Workout Plan**
0:00-5:00	Walk at a moderate pace to warm up.
5:00-6:00	Do one minute of gentle stretching for the lower body.
6:00-10:00	Repeat for 4 minutes straight: Walk for 20 seconds. Jog for 20 seconds. Run for 20 seconds.
10:00-12:00	Walk fast. Big arms, big strides.
12:00-18:00	Repeat for 6 minutes straight: Walk for 20 seconds. Jog for 20 seconds. Run for 20 seconds.
18:00-20:00	Walk fast and finish with a slow walk for a few minute OR continue and repeat the whole workout for an intense 40 minute total burn.

The Healthy Lifestyle Solution 3: Sleep Well

A healthy lifestyle would not be complete without healthy sleep habits. Getting too little sleep or having interrupted or disturbed sleep contributes to our unhealthy, destructive lifestyles. To turn that around, we must develop good sleep patterns: falling asleep, maintaining sleep, and waking renewed and refreshed.

I'm sure you can relate to the experience of wanting nothing more than to lie down and sleep. Maybe it was a late-night or maybe your child was sick during the night. Whatever the case may be, our bodies need good, quality sleep. The desire for sleep can be powerful. Sleeping well energizes and lack of sleep has the exact opposite effect.

The following ten tips can help you achieve sleep and the benefits it provides. These tips are intended for "typical" adults, but not necessarily for children or persons experiencing medical problems. Lack of adequate sleep over an extended period is a cause for concern. If you are unable to regulate your sleep, even after following guidelines like those I suggest below, you may need to consult a physician.

Dr. Karen's Top Ten Guidelines to The Healthy Lifestyle Solution 3 - Sleep Well

Solution 3, Tip 1: Create a calm sleep environment.

Have you ever gone to a spa for a nice, relaxing massage? If so, I'm sure you noticed the quiet, soft atmosphere. The peaceful music playing softly in the background. The slight smell of spice or flowers. The quiet manner in which you were addressed.

The spa purposefully creates an environment conducive to relaxation. Being able to relax and feel a sense of peace ensures we will have an enjoyable experience and will want to return again.

Our bedrooms should produce a similar feeling. Arrange your bedroom in a manner to produce in you a sense of relaxation and peace. Make it a place conducive to sleep: cool, quiet, dark, and comfortable. Eliminate anything that might interrupt or disrupt your sleep. Your partner's sleep habits such as snoring may interfere with your sleep. If so, find a solution. Wear earplugs. If it is too light, buy a pair of eye shades. Be sure your bedroom feels comfortable and invites sleep.

Solution 3, Tip 2: Maintain a regular bed and wake time schedule including weekends.

You may have heard of circadian rhythms or the circadian clock. Our bodies naturally pass through various stages throughout the day. The part of the circadian rhythms that are important with regards to sleep are the natural cycle of sleep and wakefulness.

Although it is so simple we may not think about it, our bodies follow a pattern of wakefulness during the day when it is light and sleep during the night when there is no light. It is a natural and stable pattern.

We can improve our sleep habits when we follow a pattern of waking at a certain time and going to bed at a certain, regular time. Establishing a pattern encourages that pattern. In other words, when we consistently wake at the same time and lie down for sleep at the same time, our bodies fall into a pattern.

We tend to change our pattern during the weekends when we stay up longer and sleep in longer. Disrupting an established sleep cycle on the weekends can disrupt our sleep.

Solution 3, Tip 3: Establish a bedtime ritual.

We can improve our sleep quality by establishing a bedtime routine. Doing the same thing consistently tends to produce consistent results. If we train our bodies to prepare for bed in a consistent way, our bodies will learn to expect sleep.

There are activities that may cause excitement or anxiety. These types of activities should be avoided prior to bedtime. I recommend that your bedtime routine consist of activities that relax and calm the body in preparation for sleep. Some of my clients like to relax in a warm bath or listen to calming music. Remember the spa? Be sure your bedtime routine contributes to a relaxing feeling.

Solution 3, Tip 4: Avoid eating a heavy meal within 3 hours of bedtime.

We discussed this already, but it is important. Let's reiterate. Eating a big meal or drinking before bedtime can disrupt your sleep or cause you not to fall asleep easily. You want to allow your body to relax and prepare for sleep.

If you are eating or drinking before bed, the body has to expend energy to digest. You want to sleep, but your body is still breaking down your dinner or midnight snack. Begin to develop a habit of not eating for two to three hours prior to your bedtime.

Solution 3, Tip 5: Engage in physical activity every day.

It is interesting how each of the lifestyle factors influence and impact the others. Most of the lifestyle factors in *The Healthy Lifestyle Solution* contribute to well being in more ways than one. Regular physical activity can help improve sleep and sleep habits. People who are in good physical condition tend to fall asleep more easily as well as sleep more soundly during the night.

There is one consideration I'll mention. The best time of day for exercise is different for everyone. I love to start my day with exercise. For some of us, working out later is better due to family and work commitments. I find exercising too close to bedtime keeps me awake, yet others find it relaxes them. Conduct your own experiment. The key is to find the time that works best for you, and do it!

Solution 3, Tip 6: Be cautious when using prescription medication and over-the-counter products.

Prescription medications can interfere with established sleep patterns. Some over-the-counter medications can even alter your sleep. It is best to ask your pharmacist what effects any medication may have on your sleep.

Solution 3, Tip 7: Sleep on a comfortable mattress and pillows.

It's important to sleep on a comfortable and supportive mattress. Usually a mattress lasts for 8 to 10 years after which a new one should be purchased. Be sure you are using a pillow that supports your head and neck properly and invites sleep. You can make the rest of your sleep space comfortable as we discussed earlier. Keeping your bed-mattress, sheets, and pillows-clean can reduce allergens.

Solution 3, Tip 8: Avoid stimulants before bedtime.

One common stimulant is caffeine which is found in soda, coffee, and chocolate. Products containing caffeine affect our bodies. You are likely aware of the little "high" that you receive from a cup of coffee or soda. These products can linger in the body for up to five hours. Consuming caffeine prior to bedtime can disrupt sleep. You may not think that the soda you drink before bedtime affects you at all, but it certainly isn't contributing to good sleep habits.

Smoking cigarettes is a major health risk. There are so many reasons not to smoke. However, I'll confine my comments to the topic at hand: sleep. Nicotine is a stimulant and as such must be avoided before bedtime. Smoking before lying down at night (even 3 or 4 hours before) can make falling asleep more difficult. If you are considering quitting, you now have one more good reason to stop. Nicotine is bad for your sleeping health.

Alcohol is another substance to avoid prior to bedtime. It too causes disruptions in sleep patterns and may cause you to have difficulty falling or remaining asleep.

Solution 3, Tip 9: Remove the TV from the bedroom.

Remember the circadian rhythms? Light naturally leads to wakeful-ness. When we sit in front of the TV and have all that light and action bombarding us, we are encouraging wakefulness when we want to induce sleep. It's not just the light but also the stimulation from loud sound and often negative images.

Have you ever noticed that the news gets worse as the day goes on? Let's not confuse our bodies; turn off the TV before bed. Television does not belong in your bedtime routine.

Solution 3, Tip 10: Use a sleep diary.

Keeping a sleep diary serves two purposes. First, recording when you can and cannot fall asleep or when you can or cannot stay asleep may help you discover what thoughts or food or activities keep you from enjoying the rest you need. Tracking sleep and sleep-related patterns can help you change your sleeping environment or your bedtime routine to better prepare you for sleep.

Second, you have a record of your sleep patterns should you need to visit a sleep specialist. It is possible that persistent sleep problems are related to some other health issue. If you continue to have difficulty in this area, consider seeing a sleep specialist who can help you deter-mine if there is a problem.

The Healthy Lifestyle Solution 4: Digestive Health

An important and often overlooked purpose of the digestive tract is to extract the available nutrients from the food we consume. It is only af-ter we've eaten a food that the body can utilize whatever nutrients the food contained. This marvelous system provides the means whereby we benefit from the nutrients and eliminate the rest.

Healthy digestion is essential for good health. Promoting digestive wellness in our bodies can lead to improved health because our digestion influences so many aspects of our overall well being.

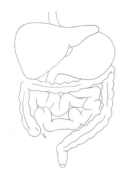

Unfortunately, too many of us suffer from some type of digestive problem. These issues range from mild problems such as indigestion to serious and life-threatening conditions like colon cancer. Poor digestive health can lead to other problems, illnesses, or disease. In fact, Eastern Medicine considers the abdomen and other digestive organs as central to health.

When our lives are in disarray, it can manifest as digestive problems. When there are digestive problems, they can manifest in other areas of the body. Digestive health is a major contributing factor to our overall well-being.

Dr. Karen's Top Ten Guidelines to The Healthy Lifestyle Solution 4 : Digestive Wellness

Solution 4, Tip 1: Remove processed foods.

By now, you are well aware of the dangers of processed and refined foods. The very process of refinement, ironically enough, often takes the nutrition out of the whole foods. These refined foods can tax the digestive tract. The more we consume these processed foods, the more taxed our digestive system becomes. By reducing or eliminating the amount of refined food and eating real, unprocessed food, we can make a significant change in our digestive health. These real foods include things such as seasonal vegetables and fruits, whole grains, nuts and seeds.

Solution 4, Tip 2: Have a diet rich in fiber.

We all know we need to eat foods that contain dietary fiber. But why? Fiber plays a vital role in digestive health. It is like the body's maid service. It needs to come through to clean up the mess. Fiber moves through the digestive tract and cleans as it goes. It scrapes debris such as waste matter, undigested bits of food, bacteria, and dead cells from the tract that would otherwise build up and cause problems.

It is commonly accepted in today's world that eating high-fiber foods protects against constipation and other digestive issues like irritable bowel syndrome.

Daily Reference Intakes (DRIs) for fiber in grams per day is 25g for adult women under 50 and 21g for adult women over 50. Adult men under 50 need 38g and adult men over 50 need 30g. Dietary fiber refers to the part of plant cell walls that is indigestible. All vegetables, fruits, whole grains, legumes, nuts and seeds contain fiber. The fiber content of a food is listed on the Nutrition Facts food label.

Our modern diet often lacks sufficient fiber. Here are some benefits of fiber, according to Mayo Clinic.

- Helps you maintain a healthy weight because food containing fiber makes you feel fuller for longer.
- Helps to regulate blood sugar levels by slowing down the absorption rate of sugars.
- Helps regulate bowel movements and avoid constipation.
- Helps lower the bad cholesterol levels which helps your heart health ("Dietary fiber: essential," 2012).

Solution 4, Tip 3: Incorporate probiotics into your diet.

As I explained in chapter 3, the gut is home to more living microorganisms than we can count. Remember that bacteria isn't always bad. In fact, much of the bacteria in our gut is essential for digestive health. The good bacteria actually helps to control the amount of bad bacteria which can only contribute to good health.

One substance you may have heard of, probiotics, is instrumental in maintaining or regulating the balance between the good and the bad bacteria present in the gut. Since many of us have some sort of imbalance in the digestive tract, these little bacteria become very important.

When you've eaten yogurt, you've probably noticed that it contains "live cultures." That may not sound like a good thing, but in fact it is a very good thing. Probiotics are these live cultures and they actually act much like our own intestinal flora.

So what do they do, you may ask? They help keep us healthy. Again, part of digestion is extracting the nutrients from food and breaking down the food for use by the body. Probiotics can help the body absorb nutrients better; they may even help break down lactose which causes many people problems. I've already mentioned that yogurt contains these live cultures but they are also found in fermented foods such as sauerkraut.

Solution 4, Tip 4: Stay hydrated.

Water is our life source, yet so many of us walk around dehydrated. With so many other beverage choices such as liquid sugar, too many of us neglect this nutrient that our bodies depend upon. We do so at our own peril. Too little water in the digestive tract means poorer elimination of waste matter. Waste matter absorbs water as it moves through the digestive tract. The water moistens the matter and makes it easier to pass.

I'd like to mention that some common beverages actually dehydrate the body in that they draw water out. These are coffee, soda, and alcohol. Replace these drinks with water. Water helps the digestive process and is absolutely necessary for good digestive health.

Solution 4, Tip 5: Reduce intake of fried, fattening foods.

We all like to lessen our workload whenever possible. One simple and direct way to lessen the stress (or workload) we place on our digestive system is to reduce the amount of high-fat foods we consume. I love french fries as much as the next person in the drive through, but I recognize just how burdensome fattening, greasy foods can be on the body.

These foods are more difficult to digest, and cutting back on them will reduce the workload of the digestive system. Cutting back on high-fat foods can help improve our digestive health.

Solution 4, Tip 6: Stop smoking and avoid excessive caffeine.

I know that I've said it before, but so many of the factors that contribute to or take away from our health do so in many ways. We know smoking and excess caffeine are bad for our health. But did you know that one way in which they are detrimental to our health is via digestion?

Things like cigarettes and caffeinated beverages can disrupt the workings of the digestive system and may lead to other problems such heartburn or ulcers. Again, there are many reasons to avoid these damaging substances. Our digestive health is simply one more to add to the growing list.

Solution 4, Tip 7: Exercise regularly.

Exercise can also contribute to good digestive health. When we engage in regular, consistent exercise, we help food move through the digestive system more regularly. The digestive tract consists of muscles. These muscles work better when we exercise.

A second reason exercise can be so beneficial to the digestive system rests with weight. Maintaining a healthy weight or losing excess weight carries with it the added benefit of improving digestive health. I always encourage my clients to incorporate even mild exercise into their daily routine to take advantage of the digestive benefits of physical activity.

Solution 4, Tip 8: Manage stress.

The question is not whether we feel stress, but how we manage the stress we feel. When we feel stressed or anxious, we cause our digestive system to work much harder. Remember those muscles we just mentioned, they constrict under stress. Learning to incorporate stress-relieving activities into our daily routine, can relieve some of the stress that we unnecessarily place on our bodies and facilitate the digestive system to function more effectively. We will discuss stress management more in depth shortly.

Solution 4, Tip 9: Eat small, frequent meals.

I have found that many of my clients who eat small meals more frequently improve their digestive health. When we eat large meals we put more stress on the digestive tract.

A good example is a huge Thanksgiving meal. Part of the sleepiness we feel after that meal is because our digestive system has to work so hard. It must use all available energy to digest the food. By eating small, frequent meals throughout the day, we utilize our energy more effectively.

Solution 4, Tip 10: Don't rush eating and chew your food

Sometimes we think of the mouth as just the place that we taste our food. However, it is actually the place where digestion begins. The mouth contains glands which contain enzymes whose purpose is to breakdown food and prepare it for the stomach. We often take large

bites and only chew the food a few times
before swallowing and sending it on its way.

We are doing our bodies a disservice when
we eat like that. Instead, we can aid the digestive process by chewing food thoroughly.

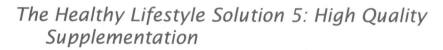

It may take some time to get used to chewing
your food more, but chewing your food to a
mushy consistency can go a long way to help
the body digest more efficiently. When we eat
too fast, we risk the build-up of undigested food that can rot in the gut.
So, slow down and chew your food. Your body will thank you for it.

The Healthy Lifestyle Solution 5: High Quality Supplementation

There is a philosophy out there that believes we can receive all of the
nutrients our bodies need through eating nutritious food. That is a
misconception. Time and again, studies show that inadequate levels
of vitamins and minerals are associated with higher risks of developing
varying chronic illnesses.

I could outline an exhaustive list of what Vitamin D or antioxidants
do to protect against chronic disease, but that is not the focus of this
book. Instead, I will recommend an article that does just that. A scientific review published in the June 19, 2002 issue of the Journal of the
American Medical Association (JAMA), notes that vitamin deficiencies
have been associated with many chronic illnesses.

Dr. Karen's Top Ten Guidelines to The Healthy Lifestyle Solution 5: Why Take High Quality Supplements

Solution 5, Tip 1: Insufficient nutrients in our food.

I cannot stress enough just how important eating nutritious food is
for our health. Having said this, I also must acknowledge that the
food we eat today, even when we are trying to eat well, is often highly
processed, may be genetically modified, and is often prepared in such
a way that destroys much of the nutritional content.

We know the benefits of consuming adequate amounts of vitamins, minerals, and antioxidants, and it is just good sense to add to an already healthy diet.

Solution 5, Tip 2: Digestive disorders.

Remember that the digestive tract extracts nutrients from the foods that we consume. We also know that our digestive systems are not always up to par. In fact, as stated previously, many of us suffer from some digestive disorder whether large or small.

The combination of a less than optimal food and a less than optimal digestive system necessitates high-quality supplementation.

Solution 5, Tip 3: Poor food preparation.

We live in a time when everything is fast. We use instant oatmeal instead of traditional oatmeal. We go through a drive through instead of preparing food at home. Many of us use a microwave oven much more often than a conventional oven. The very ways in which we prepare our food can be reducing its nutritive value.

We've established that processing food as we do so often in our modern cultures, removes nutrients that would otherwise have been present. For example, when brown rice is processed and converted to white rice, the fiber is removed as well as the most of the nutrients.

I teach my clients that good food preparation does not have to be hard or time-consuming. The key is to have a plan and to prepare as much as possible ahead of time. I sit down on Sunday and plan the meals for my family for the next week. Then I can shop for the whole week and be prepared. Weekly planning has saved me much time and stress as well as helped me avoid fast-food decisions on the run. I even started a blog of my own cooking to help my clients with healthy and easy food preparation tips because they expressed to me how important this topic was to them.

Solution 5, Tip 4: Environmental toxins.

Our modern way of life comes with certain side effects. One of those side effects is environmental toxins. It seems fairly obvious that these toxins are not healthful to the body even if the extent to which they harm us remains to be determined. Again, my purpose is not to enumerate the many toxins and what dangers each poses, rather to see as a whole the change in the environment that contributes to a need for a change in nutrient intake.

Our cells have to work harder and are under more stress due to these toxins than in previous generations. Our bodies need more nutrients to combat these toxins of which we may or may not even be aware.

Solution 5, Tip 5: Obesity.

This topic relates to the previous topic because fat is a great toxic waste dump. Fat stores toxins. Remember toxins are foreign to the body and the body often wraps the toxin in a nice protective layer of fat and stores it away.

Even releasing weight or reducing the size of the fat cells squeezes toxins out of the cell and into the bloodstream. Nutrients are the soldiers that combat these toxins.

Solution 5, Tip 6: Stress.

Here we are visiting the ever-present topic of stress again. We will be looking at stress closely in the next lifestyle factor, but I'll make a quick comment about it here. Stress saps our energy and depletes the body of nutrients. Like a vigorous workout, stress can exhaust the body's nutrients. Unfortunately, stress is part of our lives. Managing stress and providing our bodies with more than adequate nutrients becomes imperative.

Solution 5, Tip 7: Sleep deprivation.

It should become clear that we are either depleting our nutrient stores or supplying them based on our choices. Like stress, sleep deprivation can tax our nutrient supply. When our bodies have to compensate for inadequate sleep, we lose vital nutrients.

In an ideal world, we'd all get at least eight hours of uninterrupted, peaceful sleep. In reality, a huge portion of the population has some kind of sleep issues. The fact of the matter is that getting adequate sleep every night is not likely. We can minimize the damage by stocking our nutrient supplies.

Solution 5, Tip 8: Chronic dieting.

I think the term chronic dieting aptly describes the obsession our culture has with dieting. It does resemble disease. There are so many diets out there whose primary goal is losing weight, whatever the cost. Often the cost is nutrition.

It is not uncommon for a person who is dieting to actually be mal-nourished. We must be more careful in our approach to maintaining a healthy weight and releasing extra pounds. Our habit of chronic dieting increases our need for adequate nutrients.

Solution 5, Tip 9: Normal aging.

In many respects, the golden years may not be quite as golden as we might hope.

Aging really means our bodies don't produce, replicate, utilize, or work as well as they did in younger days. Aging, like other factors discussed here, necessitates greater nutritional care. We are all in the same boat here. We are getting older each day, and each day our need for high quality nutritional supplementation increases.

Solution 5, Tip 10: Athletic performance.

If you are an athlete, you need to regularly supply your body with nutrients because you are depleting them at a quicker rate than most. While it is true that exercise is good for the body and must be a part of a healthy lifestyle, there are consequences to expending that energy.

The body needs nutrients to allow the body to exercise and to recu-perate from the effects of exercise itself. Given the hectic, stressful culture we live in, nutritional supplementation just makes good sense.

The Healthy Lifestyle Solution 6: Destress Your Life

Stress is all around us. Try as we might, reducing it can be difficult if not impossible. Learning to reduce the stress we feel and managing the stress we can't eliminate can contribute exponentially to our health and quality of life.

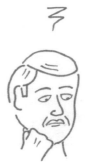

I love working with my clients in this particular area. I find most people feel unnecessary amounts of stress. Yes, it surrounds us, but there are ways to truly reduce our stress load and lift our burdens. We must recognize that there are methods to systematically lessen stress and its potentially devastating effects on our health.

I want to share with you the techniques my clients and I use to destress our lives. Try these stress-management techniques. If you need more help, don't be ashamed to ask. Sometimes the stress that causes us to engage in unhealthy behaviors is so powerful that we need outside help to get back on track.

Dr. Karen's Top Ten Guidelines to The Healthy Lifestyle Solution 6: Destress Your Life

Solution 6, Tip 1: Identify your stressors.

There are triggers that cause us to feel stress. What is stressful for one person may not be stressful for another. I cannot imagine driving a taxi in New York City. That would cause me stress. However, I am comfortable standing in front of an audience and speaking. For someone else, public speaking may send him or her over the edge.

My point is stressors are an individual thing. Find out what causes you stress. Is it thinking about having enough money to pay the bills, or is it stressing about how to spend the extra money you have? Pinpointing the situations, the topics, or people who add stress to your life is the first step to eliminating or managing that stressor.

Solution 6, Tip 2: Practice self-care.

It may sound strange to some of you, but taking care of ourselves is a necessary skill. You may be great at taking care of others--kids, parents, spouse, neighbors, friends--but lousy at taking care of you. Believe it or not, caring for yourself can improve your well-being.

Take this Self-Care Mini Assessment by answering Yes or No to each of the following:

1. ____ I exercise regularly.
2. ____ I have a way to relax that keeps me feeling centered.
3. ____ I eat healthy food that is good for me.
4. ____ I set regular time aside for solitude and silence.
5. ____ I get the sleep I need to feel fully rested.
6. ____ I spend time with friends that I truly care about.
7. ____ My home is well organized.
8. ____ I enjoy my work.
9. ____ I am able to let go of control.
10. ____ Overall, I have a positive attitude to life.

These are some tough questions. If you answered with 0 to 4 Yes's –
Hang in there. Awareness is the first step. Recognizing self care as a
priority can help you make a positive change.

If you answered yes to 5 to 7 of the questions, you are getting there.

Those of you who answered 8-10 questions in the affirmative, congrat-
ulations! You've made self-care a priority.

Solution 6, Tip 3: Take a deep breath.

You've probably been given this advice before. When we need to
relax, we can take in a nice, deep breath. Filling our lungs supplies
the body with much-needed oxygen. Ironically, when we feel stress
we tend to hold our breath instead.

Breathing deeply calms the body and mind. Taking deep breaths
causes us to slow down and to think more rationally. At times, we
react inappropriately to a stressful situation. The minute or two it takes
to breathe deeply may keep us from making matters worse.

Solution 6, Tip 4: Commit to a food/feeling diary.

Too often, our stress and our emotions influence our eating, and not
for the better. Part of distressing our lives is to separate our emotional
needs from our physical ones. Women especially tend to allow their
emotions to dictate their diet. After coaching thousands of men and
women to better wellness, I've learned just how important it can be to

BREATHING TECHNIQUES

Breathing correctly isn't as easy as it sounds. Here is a technique to help you learn to breathe deeply for stress management. It consists of three parts. Practice the three parts separately and then put them all together. You will find it relaxing.

Part One

- Sit as tall as possible.
- Exhale fully as you contract the abdominal wall and press it against your spine.
- Inhale (through your nose) as the lower abdomen expands.
- Note: While learning this breath it helps to place one of your hands on your lower abdomen to help you feel it expand.
- Exhale (through your nose) as the lower abdomen contracts and presses against the spine.

Part Two

1. Place your hands on either side of your rib cage with your thumb toward your back and your fingers in front (like putting your hands on your hips, only higher).
2. As you inhale, feel the movement expand the rib cage and push your fingers away from each other.
3. As you exhale, feel the rib cage contract and the fingers move toward each other.

Part Three: Putting it All Together

1. As you begin to inhale, feel your abdomen expand.
2. As more air enters your lungs, feel the expansion ascend through the ribs and then finally allow the collarbone to float up. You have engaged all three parts: lower abdomen, chest, and collar bones.
3. When you begin to exhale, let your collar bones begin to fall first. Then as you continue exhaling, allow your chest to deflate as the lower abdomen contracts.
4. As you become more comfortable with this breathing technique, begin to slow down both the inhalation and the exhalation.

address the idea of emotional eating. I often ask my clients to use a food/feeling diary to document when they desire unhealthful foods. I ask them to do the following:

Each time you choose to eat something, write down information as suggested in the following chart.

Look at patterns or trends that relate to your use of food to numb or change your emotional state.

Practice delaying food consumption in order to allow yourself to sit with your feelings longer.

Time of day	Food item eaten	Food item desired	How you felt prior to eating	How you felt after eating
___	___	___	___	___
___	___	___	___	___
___	___	___	___	___

Once we begin to identify the emotions that are driving our actions, we can stop ourselves from acting based off of a negative emotion or stress trigger.

Solution 6, Tip 5: Practice mindfulness.

Have you ever gone about your day and noticed that you are just going through the motions? Your mind is elsewhere and you couldn't even say where? Taking control of our thoughts and what we spend our time thinking about is an important step to destressing our lives. Developing the practice of mindfulness or awareness helps us slow down and utilize more of our own innate intelligence and sensitivity.

There are many ways to incorporate mindfulness into your life, so that it becomes your regular daily practice. Take time every morning to slow down and prepare for the day. When you find yourself going and going, pause a moment.

The adage, "Stop and smell the roses" isn't just a nice phrase. It can be a way of life.

Solution 6, Tip 6: Dare to say no.

Sometimes we bring much of our stress upon ourselves because we don't know when to say no. Whether it is obligation we feel towards others or a need to be needed, sometimes we take on more than we can bear.

> **MINDFUL EATING EXERCISE**
>
> Mindful eating helps you experience more fully the taste, texture, and temperature of food. It helps you become aware of how, when, and why you nourish yourself. It helps you handle food and dietary issues at a more conscious level.
>
> To practice mindful eating when you sit down to eat, begin by slowing down mentally.
>
> Take three slow, deep breaths and remind yourself to enjoy a moment of mindfulness.
>
> Smile and express gratitude for the food you have to nourish you.
>
> Take a moment to notice the color and appearance of the food.
>
> Give gratitude for the cook—yourself, included.
>
> For the first bite, chew your food fifteen to twenty times. How does it feel? How does the food taste? Do you feel you are being nourished?

I love to help others. My job is to help others. However, there does come a time when I have to recognize that there is no more room on my plate. Before adding more, I need to eliminate something else. Don't overburden yourself trying to do it all. Learn your limits and say no when you can't do it or when trying to do it will do more harm than good.

Solution 6, Tip 7: Get a good night's rest.

We've discussed the importance of healthy sleep habits as part of a healthy lifestyle. Getting a good night's rest can help us manage our stress better. Cortisol is an important hormone that is connected with our sleep patterns.

Too little sleep can cause stress and elevate cortisol. Too much cortisol can disrupt our ability to sleep deeply. That is not a good thing. Too little sleep is a common way we cause imbalance in our lives. Go to bed and get some sleep.

Solution 6, Tip 8: Get moving!

Exercise is an excellent way to help reduce stress. You don't need to engage in vigorous exercise to reap the benefits. A brisk walk around the block can do so much to relieve your stress burden. Incorporating exercise into your daily life and making it a part of your lifestyle can seem virtually impossible. But it isn't.

The beautiful thing about physical activity is that it can be done inside the house just dancing to music. It can be done outside working in your garden or mowing the lawn. It can be a walk with a close friend around the neighborhood. It can be in a gym or a structured class. I would like to mention some specific reasons exercise is a stress reliever and why I enjoy it so much:

1. Exercising makes you feel good. You've heard of the runner's high.

2. Exercise stimulates the release of endorphins. These neurotransmitters are like a natural pick-me-up. The good thing is you don't have to actually run to reap this benefit. Even mild exercise can release endorphins.

3. Exercising naturally relieves stress. When I am particularly burdened by stress, a workout on the stairclimber lessens the burden. Physical activity helps relieve the tension of everyday life and replaces it with energy and optimism.

4. Exercise can improve your sleep. Sleep is often interrupted by stress or depression. Because exercise is good for both, it is also good for sleeping habits.

5. Exercising improves your mood. Exercise is a low cost, natural anti-depressant. It truly can alleviate feelings of depression and anxiety. This reason alone makes it worth the effort to get up and move.

Solution 6, Tip 9: Plan out your time and prioritize.

The feeling that we have so much to do and not enough time to do it can cause a lot of stress. It's quite challenging to learn how to manage our time and maximize our efforts. However, time management is a skill that can be learned and can help to relieve much of the unnecessary stress we feel\

We all have things we must do, things we need to do, and things we'd like to do. Learning to manage our time can allow us to accomplish the tasks that are ours.

In order to properly manage our time, we must also be able to prioritize our to do list. Not every task carries the same weight. Prioritizing simply means being able to determine which tasks must be done first and second and so on.

For me, time management and prioritizing are crucial elements to distressing my life. There are many ways to learn to manage time and to prioritize, but I have found the following three skills very helpful.

Setting Goals in alignment with your values

Knowing who you are and what values govern your beliefs, attitudes, and actions can help you set appropriate goals for your life and help you determine what your priorities are.

Prioritizing Tasks

Making a to-do list of the tasks you feel are needed and then categorizing them based on how important they are is the next step in destressing your life. When those tasks that you determine are urgent are completed first, it lifts much of the stress from your shoulders. Other important but non-urgent tasks can be dealt with next. Those tasks deemed least important will just have to wait.

Avoiding Procrastination

To put it bluntly, procrastination increases your stress levels. A great way to manage your stress is to control your propensity to procrastinate. We all do it and we all suffer for it. There are three things I like to keep in mind that help me procrastinate less.

When I have a large task, I break it up into smaller pieces. It makes it so much easier to complete an overwhelming task when bits and pieces are completed instead of feeling the entire task must be done at once. I also like to give myself short-term deadlines. Finally, I do not expect perfection of myself.

DR. KAREN'S TOP TEN FAVORITE MESSAGES TO LIVE BY

LIVE IN THE PRESENT MOMENT

Do something completely on the spur of the moment today, without thinking about past experiences or future consequences

BE GENTLE WITH YOURSELF

· Give yourself and a friend a fresh bouquet of flowers

PAY ATTENTION

Stop what you are doing and observe your surroundings

FIND THE SACRED IN EVERYDAY LIFE

Abraham Maslow wrote in R*eligions, Values and Peak-Experiences*

The great lesson from the true mystics...is that the sacred is in the ordinary, that it is to be found in one's daily life, in one's neighbors, friends, and family, in one's backyard... (1994)

PRACTICE THE ART OF CONNECTION

Write a note to a friend just to tell them how much you care

HAVE A BEGINNERS MIND

Identify one area in which you are truly a beginner

PAY ATTENTION TO SYNCHRONICITY

Share with a friend a time in your life that an amazing "coincidence" occurred that changed your life

BE OPEN TO YOUR INTUITION

Share with a friend one time when you had an insight that came to you unexpectedly

SIMPLIFY

Compile a list of excesses in your life-possessions, behaviors, ideas. Which could you do without?

LEARN SOMETHING NEW

Read an article, watch a TV program or attend a lecture on a subject you know nothing about

Solution 6, Tip 10: Reduce financial stress

> *The principles that govern prosperity are very similar to the principles that govern physical and emotional health: One's financial circumstances are seamlessly connected to one's thoughts and emotions. Once you begin to see how this works in your own life, you're on the path toward financial freedom and improved health.*

> \- Christiane Northrup (*Mother Daughter Wisdom*, p. 346)

Financial stress affects all of us in some way. I cannot solve your immediate financial stress, but I can assist you to change your relationship to money. I have completely transformed my beliefs about money. I did this by studying financial literacy and committing to reading books by Catherine Ponder, Suzie Orman, and Robert Kiyosaki that shifted my thinking about money. Randy Cage is also a great author. He went from bankruptcy to millionaire by applying the laws of prosperity. One of the biggest lessons about money has come from my direct experience and involvement as a business owner with Team Northrup. Kate Northrup says it beautifully in this quote:

> *Learning how to use your passion to serve the world and create financial freedom is one of the greatest skills you could master. And putting your work out into the world in a way that helps people and creates freedom for you has the potential to change everything - for you and the world.*

> Kate Northrup (*Money: A Love Story, A Kinder Approach to Financial Freedom*, to be published by Hay House in the fall of 2013).

The Healthy Lifestyle Solution 7: Detoxify Your Environment

Chemicals. Our bodies consist of chemicals and our environment consists of chemicals. Some chemicals are good for us and necessary for our bodies to function properly, and some chemicals are not good for us or our bodies. These not-good-for-you chemicals are often man-made substances found in modern products such as plastic and non-

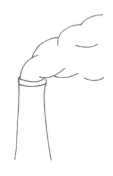

stick cookware. They can be by-products of our modern lifestyle such as car exhaust and factory pollution.

The list of potentially dangerous chemicals, or toxins, goes on for miles. These toxins have been implicated in various disorders that are on the rise. The extent to which these common toxins interfere with our health is a subject of continual investigation. That they interfere with our health is a given. My purpose, in terms of lifestyle, is to identify and reduce our exposure to daily toxins.

In chapter 3, I recommended the book called *The Healthy Home: Simple Truths to Protect Your Family from Hidden Household Dangers* by Dr. Myron Wentz and Dave Wentz. I have found this book to be extremely helpful as I made an effort to detoxify my home and my environment. Below are my favorite tips from the book.

Dr. Karen's Top Ten Guidelines to The Healthy Lifestyle Solution 7: Detoxify your Life

Solution 7, Tip 1: Start at the front door.

Leave as many toxins at the front door as possible. When you enter your home, take off your shoes. Leave the toxins on a mat beside the door rather than track them through the house.

We are in the habit of washing our hands regularly to keep bacteria at a minimum. Let's develop the equaling helpful habit of minimizing indoor toxins by leaving whatever toxins you may have gathered outside at the door.

Solution 7, Tip 2: Detoxify your containers.

Part of our modern lifestyle includes plastic. Plastic is everywhere. Many products we use contain plastic. Unfortunately this convenience comes with a price. Some plastics have been shown to release small amounts of toxins into the foods or beverages they contain.

One way to lower exposure to these toxins is to understand which plastics release more harmful toxins and which release fewer or none. If we are more aware of the products we use, we can begin to choose safer, less toxic products.

Solution 7, Tip 3: Skip the non-stick cookware.

I have thrown out my non-stick pans and have replaced them with stainless steel and glassware. The problem with non-stick cookware is that, at high temperatures, the acid used in the creation of the cookware can break down and seep into the food as we cook.

When we consume the food, we may be ingesting toxic carcinogenic substances that may be released as the acid breaks down. In an effort to minimize toxins in your home, remove non-stick pots and pans and choose iron, porcelain-coated, stainless steel, or glass pots and pans instead.

Solution 7, Tip 4: Eat pesticide-free food.

We've already established the great extent to which our food has been processed. While it is better to eat an apple than a bag of potato chips, it is better still to eat a pesticide-free apple instead of a genetically engineered apple.

Unfortunately, even healthy food can contribute to our toxic environment. Fruits and vegetables are often genetically modified and grown with high amounts of pesticides. This science allows farmers to produce more apples that withstand the elements and pests better, but the downside are the toxic chemicals that are often passed on to us.

Choosing pesticide-free food can help you take your health one step further. Not only are you choosing foods that contain vitamins, minerals, and antioxidants necessary for good health, you are also choosing to avoid certain chemicals and toxins that would otherwise be present. Also, be an informed consumer. Choose dairy products and meat that have not been enhanced with added growth hormones. Buy food that is as close to its natural state as possible.

Solution 7, Tip 5: Drink safe water.

Don't be fooled by the claim that bottled water is better for you. Instead of wasting your money on bottled water, buy a carbon pitcher or use a filter that employs reverse osmosis to limit your exposure to toxins like chlorine or lead that are found in drinking water. When you need access to water on the go, use a stainless steel, glass, or BPA-free plastic reusable container.

Solution 7, Tip 6: Skip the artificial sweeteners.

Artificial sweeteners are exactly that: artificial. They are not natural and the body often reacts adversely to them. They contain substances that are not-good-for-you substances. Rather than consume them, choose natural sweeteners such as honey (in small amounts).

Solution 7, Tip 7: Clean your indoor air quality.

We breathe air in and out all day, everyday. The air we depend upon for life contains these pesky little chemicals that aren't so good for us. Ironically, the act of staying alive exposes us to any number of toxic chemicals. Between work and school and home, we spend most of our time indoors. We may think we are safer indoors than out, but our indoor air can be polluted just like the air outside.

There are some ways we can improve the air quality in our homes. We can eliminate products that contain toxic chemicals within our homes, and we can stop smoking cigarettes and eliminate that toxin from our homes. We can also rid our homes of mold and allergens. Finally, we can choose to filter the air within our homes by using a good quality air purifying system.

Solution 7, Tip 8: Dry clean alert.

I don't have my clothes dry cleaned anymore. I've learned that products used during the dry cleaning process contain chemicals that adversely affect hormones. These types of products have been banned in places like Europe and Canada. There is an effort to have them banned in the United States as well.

If you choose to dry clean your clothes, look for a business that does not use these harmful products.

Solution 7, Tip 9: Clean greener.

Cleaning products are often a huge offender with regard to toxic chemicals. However, in today's consumer-savvy world, many companies now make products that are safe and environmentally sound. Limit the toxins in your home by choosing these chemical-free, environmentally sound products or use common household products in place of cleaners. For instance, you can use vinegar instead of bleach or use hydrogen peroxide instead of stain remover.

Solution 7, Tip 10: Purify your personal care products.

The toxic load in our personal care products such as shampoo, conditioner, face wash, and moisturizer is often overlooked. The parabens often used in producing personal care products are now believed to be a factor in some chronic illnesses.

Products like shampoos, deodorants and toothpaste can have high concentration of chemicals. Switching to preservative-free personal care products is one way in which you can detoxify your body and lifestyle.

The Healthy Lifestyle Solution 8: Create Healthy Support Systems

In the introduction of this book, I quoted Margaret Mead who said, "Never doubt that a small group of thoughtful, committed citizens can change the world." The idea that groups of people can bring about change is central to my philosophy on health and wellness. As I said before, wellness doesn't just happen.

It takes effort; sometimes it takes a lot of effort. If the root of our health concerns rests with our lifestyle choices and habits, it is the lifestyle we must address. Making long-lasting changes can be difficult. Creating healthy communities that aid you on your journey to changing your lifestyle is vital to your success.

Part of the reason I love the work I do so much is because I feel that I am helping create support systems for my clients. The role of healthy communities is often overlooked in terms of diet and exercise goals.

The people with whom we associate, the activities in which we engage, the habits we form in our interactions with our friends, family members, and co-workers often contribute to our success or failure to make our desired lifestyle changes. Through my role as coach and mentor, I've seen the necessity of creating uplifting communities built upon strong relationships.

Think for a moment about how you spend time with close friends and family members. Do you get together around a table full of less than healthy food or at a play date at the local fast food joint? Do you meet with your friends for a walk around the block or for pizza and a movie?

Consider for a moment your social interactions and how well they align with your own personal goals. Are they a match? If you are like most, the answer, sadly, is not usually.

As I speak and work with people around the country, I find many people who have formed friendships based on supporting each other. I have met friends who walk together, cook together, travel together, sew together, dance together, paint together, and, of course, shop together. These healthy, supportive friendships are the basis of creating positive change in our lives.

Making lifestyle changes like those we've discussed in this chapter can be too hard to do alone. I encourage you to create your own support network. Think of the changes you need to make to change your killer lifestyle to a lifestyle that embraces health and wellness.

Think about your interests and areas of your life where you desire support and connection. Begin to reach out to others and find like-minded people who can be part of your support as you are part of theirs.

Dr. Karen's Top Ten Guidelines to The Healthy Lifestyle Solution 8: Create Healthy Support Systems

Solution 8, Tip 1: An exercise group.

Exercise is a simple way to begin to shift your lifestyle. It is a great place to start, and what's even better is that it is easy to do with a partner. Find a friend who will walk with you or go to the gym with you. You'll find you begin to look forward to the interaction with your friend as well as the exercise.

Solution 8, Tip 2: A spiritual group.

Part of our overall well-being includes a spiritual component. Regardless of religious affiliation, we share a need for meaning and purpose. Belonging to or creating a group based on your personal spiritual meaning can help support the other lifestyle changes you want to make.

Solution 8, Tip 3: An "extended family" of neighbors.

Life can be challenging and often presents situations for which you need help. Having family around can be a comfort in that you have help available should you need it. However, many people are like me and don't live near their families. Instead I have wonderful neighbors. These neighbors have become my extended family and we provide the support to each other when life's challenges come to call.

Solution 8, Tip 4: A book club.

For me and for many people I know, reading a good book is a great way to relieve stress and form friendships. I formed my own book club where we meet once a month in different homes and discuss the book and have lots of social time.

Solution 8, Tip 5: A hiking or other outdoor activity group.

Three years ago, I bought a guidebook that showed all the great hiking trails in my community. I had no idea there were so many. I have hiked different trails with different friends and even joined a local hiking group!

Solution 8, Tip 6: A yoga class.

Meditation is a great way to relieve stress and bring balance to your life. For me yoga is a form of meditation. You can easily find videos that provide yoga routines you can share with a small group of people. Or you can find a yoga instructor and join a local class.

Solution 8, Tip 7: A hobby group.

There are networking groups for nearly every interest, hobby, or business. Wherever your interests lie, there is sure to be a local or virtual group available for you to network with others.

Solution 8, Tip 8: A cooking club.

Food plays a major role in our lives and preparing and eating good, healthy food will be a part of your new and improved lifestyle. One great way to find support in this department is to join or create a cooking club. Cooking has become a favorite pastime for many of us.

Cooking good food that is also good for us can be a fun challenge to tackle. It is even more fun when done with others.

Solution 8, Tip 9: A bike club.

Biking is a great form of exercise that also gets us out in nature. Most of us will take any excuse to get out of the office or home and go into nature. Find a local trail and others who enjoy biking (or just enjoy being outside) and ride together.

Solution 8, Tip 10: Sign up for a class!

There are so many classes you can take in your community. Look in the local community paper and see what interests you!

Join me for health's sake.

I have seen the changes that have come about in the lives of many people when they've committed to making these lifestyle changes in their own lives. I have seen people change their lives by changing their daily choices. Instead of making choices that foster disease and unhappiness, they've begun to make choices that promote the wellness and happiness they desire.

The eight lifestyle solutions I've outlined here are a blueprint to changing your killer lifestyle. Make a choice to take one small step today that will lead to making bigger changes tomorrow. Join me in creating lifestyles of wellness. Together, we can begin to change the world.

Dr. Karen's Final Words: The Ongoing Journey

With most lifestyle change, we can relapse and default back to our old habits fairly easily. A major stress in life can trigger old coping mechanisms. This program is about progress, not perfection. My own personal journey with food and sugar issues has taught me that the answer is not about deprivation. In fact, the more we deprive and restrict, the bigger the relapse. We are wired for pleasure, so it is important to add "healthy pleasures" to our daily lives.

You, like most of us, have probably had mixed results with a variety of other programs in the past. That is OK. With the tools of this program you can take back control of your life. Reaching a target weight is a great milestone, but it is not the end of the journey. Surround yourself with people who support you on your road to recovery and be aware of others who might want to sabotage your success.

Because this is a journey, reading this book is only the first step. To help you continue along your road to recovery, I've included:

1. A Checklist of all the Guidelines for *The Healthy Lifestyle Solution*.

2. A Resource Section with listings under each specific Lifestyle Factor.

3. Coaching resources for coaches who might want to use *The Healthy Lifestyle Solution* with clients.

I will leave you with a quote by Mark Twain that reminds me that change happens one step at a time. Be patient with yourself as you improve your life.

> *Habit is habit, and not to be flung out of the window by any man, but coaxed down-stairs one step at a time.*

> — *Mark Twain*

References

DesMaisons, K. (1999). *Potatoes not prozac. New York: Simon & Schuster.*

Dietary fiber: essential for a healthy diet. (2012, Nov 17). Retrieved from http://www.mayoclinic.com/health/fiber/NU00033

Fairfield, K. M., & Fletcher, R. H. (2002). Vitamins for chronic disease prevention in adults scientific review. *The Journal of the American Medical Association, 287*(23), 3116-3126. doi: 10.1001/jama.287.23.3116.

Ford, E. S. (2002). Does exercise reduce inflammation? physical activity and c-reactive protein among us adults. *Epidemiology, 13*(5), 561-568. Retrieved from http://www.jstor.org/stable/3703940.

Maslow, A. (1994). *Religions, values, and peak experiences. New York: Penguin Group.* Retrieved from http://www.nostrajewellery.org/files/Abraham-H.-Maslow-Religions,-Values-and-Peak-Experiences.pdf

Northrup, C. (2006). *Mother-daughter wisdom.* (p. 346). New York: Bantam Dell.

Northrup, K. (2013). *Money: a love story, a kinder approach to financial freedom. San Diego: Hay House. In press.*

Solution Summary

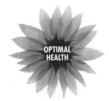

What follows are listings for each collection of guidelines ("tips") in the eight sections of Chapter 5's The Healthy Lifestyle Solution. I provide these to you as an easy reference that you might check-off as you focus on each guideline.

FOOD PLAN

1. _____ Consider jump starting your food plan.
2. _____ Eat protein and "whole" carbohydrates with every meal.
3. _____ Eat every 3-4 hours to keep your blood sugar and insulin levels balanced.
4. _____ Eat small snacks with protein – such as handful of nuts.
5. _____ Beware of nighttime eating.
6. _____ Always eat breakfast.
7. _____ Always have low-glycemic snacks available.
8. _____ Focus on low-glycemic foods and make slow-burning vegetables the foundation of your meal.
9. _____ Focus on anti-inflammatory foods – wild caught fish, purple and red berries, dark green leafy vegetables.
10. _____ Keep a food/feeling journal.

RESTORE PHYSICAL ACTIVITY

1. _____ See your doctor before you start any exercise program.
2. _____ Maximize the benefit of your exercise routine.
3. _____ Set realistic goals.
4. _____ Use the buddy system.
5. _____ Choose activities you like.
6. _____ Try a pedometer.
7. _____ Take the stairs.
8. _____ Plan exercise into your day.
9. _____ Reward yourself.
10. _____ Be prepared.

SLEEP WELL

1. _____ Create a calm sleep environment.
2. _____ Maintain a regular bed and wake time schedule including weekends.
3. _____ Establish a bedtime ritual.
4. _____ Avoid eating a heavy meal within 3 hours of bedtime.
5. _____ Engage in physical activity every day.
6. _____ Be cautious when using prescription medication and over-the-counter products.
7. _____ Sleep on a comfortable mattress and pillows.
8. _____ Avoid stimulants before bedtime.
9. _____ Remove the TV from the bedroom.
10. _____ Use a sleep diary.

DIGESTIVE HEALTH

1. _____ Remove processed foods.
2. _____ Have a diet rich in fiber.
3. _____ Incorporate probiotics into your diet.
4. _____ Stay hydrated.
5. _____ Reduce intake of fried, fattening foods.
6. _____ Stop smoking and avoid excessive caffeine.
7. _____ Exercise regularly.
8. _____ Manage stress.
9. _____ Eat small, frequent meals.
10. _____ Don't rush eating and chew your food.

WHY CHOOSE HIGH QUALITY SUPPLEMENTATION?

1. _____ Insufficient nutrients in our food.
2. _____ Digestive disorders.
3. _____ Poor food preparation.
4. _____ Environmental toxins.
5. _____ Obesity.
6. _____ Stress.
7. _____ Sleep deprivation.
8. _____ Chronic dieting.
9. _____ Normal aging.
10. _____ Athletic performance.

DESTRESS YOUR LIFE

1. _____ Identify your stressors.
2. _____ Practice self-care.
3. _____ Take a deep breath.
4. _____ Commit to a food/feeling diary.
5. _____ Practice mindfulness.
6. _____ Dare to say no.
7. _____ Get a good night's rest.
8. _____ Get moving!
9. _____ Plan out your time and prioritize.
10. _____ Reduce financial stress.

DETOXIFY YOUR ENVIRONMENT

1. _____ Start at the front door.
2. _____ Detoxify your containers.
3. _____ Skip the non-stick cookware.
4. _____ Eat pesticide-free food.
5. _____ Drink safe water.
6. _____ Skip the artificial sweeteners.
7. _____ Clean your indoor air quality.
8. _____ Dry clean alert.
9. _____ Clean greener.
10. _____ Purify your personal care products.

CREATE HEALTHY SUPPORT SYSTEMS

1. _____ An exercise group.
2. _____ A spiritual group.
3. _____ An "extended family" of neighbors.
4. _____ A book club.
5. _____ A hiking or other outdoor activity group.
6. _____ A yoga class.
7. _____ A hobby group.
8. _____ A cooking club.
9. _____ A bike club.
10. _____ Sign up for a class.

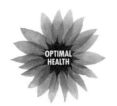

Resources

ALSO BY THE AUTHOR

Wolfe, Karen, and Deborah Kern. *Create the Body Your Soul Desires: The Friendship Solution to Weight, Energy and Sexuality. (Healing Quest, 2003).*

Wolfe, Karen. *Glycemic Index Made Easy:Top Ten Frequently Asked Questions About Glycemic Index (CD), 2012.*

Wolfe, Karen. *Medicine from the Inside Out (Audiobook). Healing Quest Publishing; 2010.*

Wolfe, Karen. *Visualizations for Healing (CD). Healing Quest Publishing; 2009.*

DR. KAREN'S FAVORITE RESOURCES
FOR
THE HEALTHY LIFESTYLE SOLUTION FACTORS

Healthy Lifestyle Solution 1: The Food Plan, Food as Medicine

DesMaisons, Kathleen. *The Sugar Addict's Total Recovery Program (Ballantine Books, 2000).*

DesMaisons, Kathleen. *Potatoes not Prozac. New York: (Simon & Schuster, 1999).*

Hyman, Mark. *The Blood Sugar Solution: The UltraHealthy Program for Losing Weight, Preventing Disease, and Feeling Great Now! (Little, Brown and Company; 2012).*

Kalina, Laura and Christian, Cheryl. *Low Glycemic Meals in Minutes (Real Life Press, 2007).*

Naparstek, Belleruth. *A Meditation to help you with Weight Loss. Audio CD (Health Journeys, 1997).*

Northrup, Christiane. *Women's Bodies, Women's Wisdom. (Bantam Books, 2010).*

Ornish, Dean. *Dr. Dean Ornish's Program for Reversing Heart Disease. (Random House, 1990).*

Robertson, Joel. *Peak Performance Living:Drug-Free Ways to Alter Your Own Brain Chemistry. (Harper Collins, 1996).*

Rosenthal, Joshua. *Integrative Nutrition. New York: (Integrative Nutrition Publishing, 2007).*

Weaver, Libby. *Accidentally Overweight*. Auckland: (Little Green Frog Publishing Ltd, 2010).

Willett, Walter. *Eat, drink, and be healthy*. New York: (Free Press, 2005).

WEBSITES

www.glycemicindex.com

I use this website to look up the specific glycemic index and glycemic load of specific foods. It also has great recipes.

www.drkarenwolfe.usana.com

Here I provide access to the 5-Day Sugar Cleanse I use myself and with my clients. Or you can order from any USANA Health Sciences Associate.

www.radiantrecovery.com

I refer my clients to this website for more information on sugar sensitivity. There are online classes and a community forum for people to participate in.

www.geneenroth.com

Geneen taught me that the way we eat is inseparable from the way we live our lives. This is a good website for emotional eating resources.

Healthy Lifestyle Solution 2: Restore Physical Activity

Kaehler, Kathy. *Celebrity Workouts: How to Get a Hollywood Body in Just 30 Minutes a Day*.(Broadway Books 2005).

Kaehler, Kathy. *Total Body Workout: 6 Ten Minute Workouts*. DVD 2009.

Loube, Brenda. *You Can Play*. (HTA Books, 2011).

Lusk, Julie. *Desktop Yoga* (Perigee Trade, 1998).

Peeke, Pam. *Body for Life for Women: A Woman's Plan for Physical and Mental Transformation*, (Rodale Books, 2005).

Rosas, Carlos and Debbie. *The Nia Technique: The High-Powered Energizing Workout that Gives You a New Body and a New Life*. (Three Rivers Press, 2005).

WEBSITES

www.fitness.gov

This is the President's Council on Fitness, Sports, and Nutrition.

www.acsm.org

This is the American College of Sports Medicine.

Healthy Lifestyle Solution 3: Sleep Well

Dement, William. *The Promise of Sleep: A Pioneer in Sleep Medicine Explores the Vital Connection Between Health, Happiness, and a Good Night's Sleep*. (Dell, 2000).

Maas, James. *Sleep for Success! Everything You Must Know About Sleep But are Too Tired to Ask.* (AuthorHouse, 2011).

Naparstek, Belleruth. *Health Journeys: A Meditation to Help You with Healthful Sleep* [Audio CD] Health Journeys, 2000.

WEBSITES

www.sleepfoundation.org

This is the National Sleep Foundation.

Healthy Lifestyle Solution 4: Digestive Health

Gershon, Michael. *The Second Brain: A Groundbreaking New Understanding of Nervous Disorders of the Stomach and Intestine* (Harper Collins, 1999).

Lipski, Elizabeth. *Digestive Wellness: Strengthen the Immune System and Prevent Disease Through Healthy Digestion,* (McGraw-Hill; 4 edition, 2011).

Lipski. Elizabeth. *Digestive Wellness for Children: How to Strengthen the Immune System & Prevent Disease Through Healthy Digestion* (Basic Health Publications, 2006).

Healthy Lifestyle Solution 5: High Quality Supplementation

MacWilliam, Lyle. *NutriSearch Comparative Guide to Nutritional Supplements.* (Northern Dimensions, 2011).

MacWilliam, Lyle. *Comparative Guide to Children's Nutritionals.* (Northern Dimensions, 2004).

Holick, Michael. *The Vitamin D Solution: A 3-Step Strategy to Cure Our Most Common Health Problem.* (Hudson Street Press, 2010).

WEBSITES

www.usana.com

USANA Health Sciences offers state-of-the-art pharmaceutical grade vitamins and mineral supplements.

www.consumerlab.com

I use this website to research independent testing of nutritional products.

Healthy Lifestyle Solution 6: Destress your Life

Benson, Herbert. *Beyond the Relaxation Response.* (Time Life Books, 1984).

Kern, Deborah. *Everyday Wellness for Women.* (Slaton Press, 1999).

Naparstek, Belleruth. *Staying Well with Guided Imagery.* (Warner Books, 1995).

Naparstek, Belleruth. *Meditations to Relieve Stress* Audio CD (Health Journeys,(1995).

Sapolsky, Robert. *Why Zebras Don't Get Ulcers: A Guide to Stress, Stress-Related Diseases, and Coping*. (W.H.Freeman, 1998).

Schenker, Melissa and Moody, Tina. *Sweet Relief from the Everyday Narcissist*. (Live Oak Book Company, 2012).

Northrup, Kate. *Money: A Love Story, A Kinder Approach to Financial Freedom*. (In press with Hay House, Inc., 2013).

WEBSITE

www.healthjourneys.com

This is an invaluable source for guided imagery and other mind-body resources.

Healthy Lifestyle Solution 7: Detoxify your Environment

Sass, Lorna J. *Recipes from an Ecological Kitchen: Healthy Meals for You and the Planet*. (Morrow, 1992).

Wentz, Myron and Wentz, Dave. *The Healthy Home: Simple Truths to Protect Your Family from Hidden Household Dangers*. (Vanguard Press; First Trade Paper Edition edition, 2012).

Wood, Christine. *ADHD: Environmental Factors and Nutrition* (CD). 2012.

WEBSITES

www.cspinet.org

This is the Center for Science in the Public Interest (CSPI) which has great resources on environmental health.

www.drkarenwolfe.usana.com

Use this website to order safe personal care products as you phase out the use of chemicals on your body.

Healthy Lifestyle Solution 8: Create Healthy Support Systems

Ornish, Dean. *Love and Survival*. (Harper Collins, 1998).

Roth, Geneen. *When Food is Love*. (Dutton, 1989).

Roth, Geneen. *Women Food and God: An Unexpected path to Almost Everything* (Simon & Shuster, Inc., 2010).

Tate, Susan. *Wellness Wisdom: 31 Ways to Nourish Your Mind, Body, & Spirit*. (iUniverse, Inc., 2011).

WEBSITES

www.functionalmedicine.org

This is the website for the Institute of Functional Medicine. I send my clients to this website to find a functional medicine practitioner in their area. (Functional medicine focuses on the underlying causes of health and disease).

www.sanoviv.com

I send my clients to this website for specific holistic approaches to health concerns such as cancer, diabetes, allergies, and thyroid issues.

www.drweil.com

This is a great website about integrative medicine that has up-to-date articles, recipes, and search features. (Integrative medicine is a blend of many different healing philosophies).

OTHER RESOURCES

CHILDREN'S HEALTH

Northrup, Christiane with Kristina Tracy. Beautiful Girl: Celebrating the Wonders of Your Body (Hay House, Inc., 2013).

Wood, Christine. How to Get Kids to Eat Great & Love It! (KidsEatGreat, Inc. 2002).

WEBSITES

www.KidsEatGreat.com

This is a great resource to help children develop good nutritional habits, and it has great eating tips for all ages.

MEAL PLANNING

www.kathykaehler.net

I use the Sunday Set-up feature of this website to help me prepare food for my week. It saves me time and ensures I have healthy food available each week.

www.drkarenwolfe.org/the-sugar-busters

Here I have videos called Karen's Kitchen in which I prepare low-glycemic meals.

MUSIC

www.janastanfield.com

Jana's music is often referred to as heavy mental music. I use it to inspire me and uplift my audience at speaking engagements.

www.karendrucker.com

Karen's songs are inspirational, and the lyrics have very positive messages.

COACHING RESOURCES

Arloski, M. *Wellness coaching for lasting lifestyle change*. (Whole Person Associates, 2007).

Rosenberg, Marshall. *Nonviolent Communication: A Language of Life*. (PuddleDancer Press, 2003).

Whitworth, L., Kimsey-House, K., Kimsey-House, H., & Sandahl, P. *Co-active coaching: New skills for coaching people toward success in work and life.* (Davies-Black, 2007).

How to Ask Powerful Coaching Questions

A powerful question evokes clarity and action. It creates greater possibility and new learning. Powerful questions are open-ended questions that do not elicit a yes or no response. Below are examples of powerful questions that are taken from the book *Create the Body Your Soul Desires* by Dr. Wolfe and Dr. Kern, 2003.

What are you willing to do to have more energy? (This type of question helps you begin to outline an action plan based on your willingness to take action).

What would it feel like to feel better in your body? (This type of question helps you to be more specific about a vague goal).

How will you feel when you have more energy (or achieve the goal of feeling better in your body)? (This question, like the last one, helps you begin to imagine the physical sensations they will feel when you achieve your goal).

What will you hear when you have achieved your goal? (This question engages the sense of hearing. For example, the client may imagine hearing hearing comments from friends on their renewed energy level).

What will you see when you have more energy? (This question engages the sense of sight. They may see themselves engaging in their daily activities with lots of energy or completing projects they have been putting off).

How will you know when you have more energy? (This type of question helps make the goal measurable).

By when would you like to achieve this goal? (This question helps the client begin to create a time frame).

What has worked for you before? (This question helps the client realize what skills they already have).

What baby step are you willing to do in the next week to move toward this goal? (This question helps the client to get specific about the next step).

Do you need support to meet this goal? How and when will you ask for this support? (This question gets the client thinking about the need for support).

Do you know anyone or any books that could outline processes that would work for you? (This is another question to get the client to think of other sources of support).

Are you 85% sure you can achieve this goal? (This question helps the client create a plan that is do-able. If they answer "no," then they need to modify the action step so they are at least 85% sure).